AARON ROGERS

Peaceful, pain free and dignified:
palliative and end of life care for people on the autism spectrum
A guide for social care practitioners

Jill Ferguson and Val Laurie

British Library Cataloguing in Publication Data

A CIP record for this book is available from the British Library

© BILD Publications 2015

BILD Publications is the imprint of:

British Institute of Learning Disabilities
Birmingham Research Park
97 Vincent Drive
Edgbaston
Birmingham
B15 2SQ

Telephone: 0121 415 6960

E-mail: enquiries@bild.org.uk

Website: www.bild.org.uk

No part of this book may be reproduced without prior permission from the publisher, except for the quotation of brief passages for review, teaching or reference purposes, when an acknowledgement of the source must be given.

ISBN 978 1 905218 41 7

BILD Publications are distributed by:

BookSource
50 Cambuslang Road
Cambuslang
Glasgow
G32 8NB

Telephone: 0845 370 0067

Fax: 0845 370 0068

For a publications catalogue with details of all BILD books and journals e-mail enquiries@bild.org.uk or visit the BILD website www.bild.org.uk

Printed in the UK by Latimer Trend and Company Ltd, Plymouth

People with learning disabilities and people with autism want to make their own choices and decisions about the things that affect their lives. To help make this happen, BILD works to influence policy-makers and campaigns for change, and our services can help organisations improve their service design and develop their staff to deliver great support.

Contents

Forewords *by Michael Baron and Charlene Tait*   5
Preface *by Jill Ferguson*   9

Introduction   11

What is palliative care?   12
The autism spectrum   14
Meet Stephane   16
Meet the team   20

Chapter 1: Physical   25

Care planning   29
Managing symptoms and the effects of illness   35
Advance care planning   37
Support environments   40
At the end of life   45
Physical: final thoughts   48
Physical: discussion points for care teams   50
Physical: support mapping   51

Chapter 2: Psychological   53

Supporting understanding   55
Processing information   60
Emotions and feelings   62
Loss of self ability   68
Psychological: final thoughts   69
Psychological: discussion points for care teams   70
Psychological: support mapping   71

Chapter 3: **Social** — 73

- **Social support for people on the autism spectrum** — 75
- **Friends and peers on the autism spectrum** — 78
- **Family and friends** — 81
- **Support from other agencies** — 86
- **Support for care staff** — 87
- **Social: final thoughts** — 90
- **Social: discussion points for care teams** — 92
- **Social: support mapping** — 93

Chapter 4: **Spiritual** — 95

- **The search for meaning and significance in life** — 97
- **Religious and cultural customs** — 104
- **A good death** — 108
- **Spiritual: final thoughts** — 110
- **Spiritual: discussion points for care teams** — 112
- **Spiritual: support mapping** — 113

Perspectives — 115

Final thoughts — 119

Information and support — 125

References — 126

Forewords

Peaceful, pain free and dignified, in short, the good death. What in mediaeval times was called *'ars moriendi'*, the art of dying. At the age of 86, I want this for myself, but just as much I want that end of life art for people on the autism spectrum like my son. I am honoured to be asked to write this foreword to an essential (probably the first) guide to end of life care for people on the autism spectrum.

'Care' lies at the heart of the matter. For dying is a time of suffering and too often, as Dr Atul Gawande observes in his book, *Being Mortal* (2014), a struggle against *"the seemingly unstoppable momentum of medical treatment"*. In his penultimate chapter covering *"hard conversation"*, the contents itself a succinct summary of aspects of mortality, Gawande reminds us that despite outcome directed pathways of medicine, and the best technology, there is *"another kind of care"*.

But how is this most wanted of aims to be achieved, not least for people without legal capacity or with only a limited ability to make decisions about treatment? How can they anticipate, indeed imagine the end of life? Many people with autism will never have that hard conversation, relying on family and carers to interpret imperfect utterances and exceptional body language. Dr Jonathan Koffman, Kings College Hospital (London) lecturer in palliative medicine, fears that *"relatives are sometimes excluded from critical conversations about the end of the loved one's life"* (Dreaper, 2015). This guide explains how 'hard conversations' should take place. And, the subtitle notwithstanding, it is for a wider public than social care practitioners.

For myself, as father, the guide is long awaited. Parents and siblings worry about futures as we, and our kin on the spectrum, age. They will benefit from the wisdom, expertise and compassion in these pages, centred on the life and death of Stephane, a 45 year old man with pancreatic cancer, as his closing years were played out. Our anxieties, too, are well known. No one has listened as much as Jill Ferguson and Val Laurie, and spelled out the details of the best way to go. We are hugely grateful that BILD commissioned this guide with explanatory graphics to complement the text.

While the men and women first diagnosed with the complex condition or disorder were 0.45% of the population in the first statistical study in 1966, autism is now global: 2% in 2014 (US Centres for Disease Control and Prevention, 2015) or an alleged 3.5 million in the USA alone.

Whatever contemporary disagreements there may be about meaning, outcomes and place in society, so many on the spectrum are growing older and dying. Those with learning or intellectual disabilities will require the most support, the most understanding, the most care and love. So here it is.

Chapter headings preceded by an explanatory introduction are physical, psychological, social and spiritual support. The signposts for information, the support mapping templates, discussion points for care teams and the inclusive bibliography are invaluable. These show the width of the authors' study and experience and how widely they have read and absorbed the lessons of the literature of palliative care, as have the team that cared for Stephane.

No easy subject, this book is brave, necessary and timely. There is a profound connection between the search for 'meaning and significance in life' and the much desired good death. Above all the life force which even in the most disabled of individuals shines brightly through mists of incoherence should be ended with as much consent and conversation as possible in peace, free from pain and with dignity. This book explains how.

References

Dreaper, J (2015) Care of dying patients 'still inconsistent and poor'. BBC News report, 4 September. Available at: www.bbc.co.uk/news/health-34144863

Gawande, A (2014) *Being Mortal: Illness, Medicine and What Matters in the End*. London: Profile Books/Wellcome Collection.

US Centres for Disease Control and Prevention (2015) *Autism Spectrum Disorder Data and Statistics*. Available at: www.cdc.gov/ncbddd/autism/data.html

Michael Baron

There can be few things more challenging than supporting someone towards the end of their life. Within Scottish Autism, there are very few people we have had to support in this way to date, but as time goes by we know we will not be the only organisation faced with providing comfort and care to people with autism in the last days of their lives.

Such sensitive experiences are difficult and challenging for everyone involved. They are, however, important to talk about. The expectations placed on professional support staff can, at times, fail to recognise the complexity of the relationships that develop with the people we support and, in a lot of cases, sustain over many years.

The team featured in this book found it very difficult to access practical resources to guide and support them. The story they tell is of course a unique experience; however, it is also a very human experience and one that is shared with the intention of enabling others who may find they are facing a similar situation.

Within Scottish Autism we are working to develop and embed a culture of knowledge sharing among our own staff teams and with the wider community. This involves supporting and encouraging practitioners to record, reflect on and disseminate their experiences. In doing so, we can increase organisational knowledge and can also identify what constitutes ethical and effective autism practice.

As a large organisation whose mission is to enable people living with autism in Scotland through the *whole* life journey, this work feels particularly poignant. It demonstrates that we need to focus on practice that not only enables people to lead the life they wish but to end their life with dignity.

In their support of the individual who inspired this piece of work, the support team clearly demonstrated that they embody our organisational values. In developing this work Jill Ferguson, Val Laurie and their extended team have also led the way in demonstrating to others that what practitioners often view as 'just doing their job' can inspire, influence and inform the practice of their peers.

Charlene Tait

**Director of Development
Scottish Autism**

Preface

Death is not an easy subject to write about. At the early stages of identifying a working title for this practice guide, Val and I were already engaged in a lengthy debate about use of language and sharing of content for fear of insensitivity when addressing the topic of life-limiting illness and end of life care. With life comes the inevitability of death, and yet we often remain uncomfortable reflecting on this subject so sensitive and open to ethical, social and spiritual debate. The concept of life and death is profound, it is a weighty and complex subject but one which affects us all regardless of culture, beliefs, age or ability.

The writers of this practice guide work for Scottish Autism in support services for adults on the autism spectrum. The decision to start having conversations about end of life care was inspired by the experience of a team of autism support workers from Scottish Autism who supported a 48 year old man called Stephane throughout his life and ultimately his death from cancer in 2013. In addition to the expected physical, practical and emotional challenges faced when delivering care for a person at the end of their life, the impact of Stephane's autism on his thinking, understanding and response to his illness posed additional support challenges and questions. Many of these challenges had never before been experienced by the health and social care staff supporting him. Therefore we wanted to capture some of those experiences and develop a practice guide that would be a support to teams such as Stephane's, faced with delivering support to other individuals on the autism spectrum at the end of their lives. Some names and details within Stephane's story have been anonymised to protect the confidentiality of those involved. Discussions have also taken place to explore the ethical considerations of sharing the story from such a significant life event, recognising the ethics of consent and the value of reciprocal trust in the relationships between storytellers and listeners (Drumm, 2013).

The mission statement of Scottish Autism states our commitment to providing support for people on the autism spectrum 'through the whole life journey' and inevitably that will include end of life care. But to get the holistic support right for someone in their death you first have to understand what is important to them in their life. It is with a developed understanding of someone's values, beliefs and personal understanding that we *"put life into their days, not just days into their life"* (The Worldwide Palliative Care Alliance, 2014).

The Scottish Government's national action plan for palliative and end of life care advocates:

> "an approach to care which is person-centred and based on neither diagnosis or prognosis but on patient and carer needs... which recognises the diversity of life circumstances of people who will need palliative and end of life care."
>
> (Scottish Government, 2008)

Autism is a neuro-developmental condition that creates differences in the way a person typically communicates, interacts and processes information about the world around them. The way that affects the person will vary significantly from one individual to another. Therefore to provide support to the person in any area of their life involves an acknowledgement that the person may have an atypical or unique perspective on aspects of their life – and also on their death – that we must respect and endeavour to understand.

The team that supported Stephane at the end of his life understood what was important to him, and ensured that Stephane the individual was at the forefront of all decisions taken regarding his palliative and end of life care. In her book *Autism and Spirituality* Olga Bogdashina writes of two types of knowledge: science as material knowledge; and wisdom relating to personal growth and learning, understanding *"who we truly are"* (Bogdashina, 2013). To deliver exemplary and appropriate palliative care to any person involves a coming together of science and wisdom, and an acknowledgement that peace at the end of life comes not just from medical intervention and symptom control but from an understanding of who we are and what is important to us in life.

The team supporting Stephane showed wisdom, commitment and compassion in their care of him both in life and in death, and the authors of this practice guide would like to thank both them and Stephane's family for their support and inspiration.

Jill Ferguson

Services Manager
Scottish Autism

Introduction

This resource is based on the experience of a team of individuals providing support to Stephane, a person on the autism spectrum. It charts his journey through palliative and end of life care, from his diagnosis with terminal pancreatic cancer, to his death in 2013.

Stephane's story

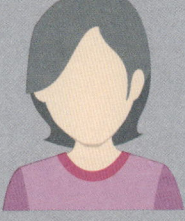
Marian
Mum

> Stephane was diagnosed with terminal cancer in 2010. I couldn't believe it, I had no idea he was so unwell. But we heard it from the specialist in Aberdeen, then got a second opinion from the specialist in Edinburgh, they couldn't both be wrong. I just thought to myself, what has caused this?

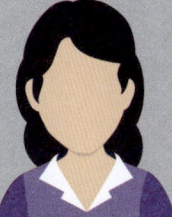
Kirsty
Keyworker

> When we went to see the specialist they told us Stephane had three to six months to live. We were devastated, we had no idea it was so bad. We knew something was wrong and had pushed for an appointment but he was still getting up every day and following his usual routine, taking part in his usual activities, and he continued to do so following his diagnosis. After about a year with very little change we started to question their diagnosis. He'd been very stable for such a long time and everything we'd read and been told said that he'd deteriorate quickly. We pushed the consultant to have him scanned again to see how his tumour was progressing. Unfortunately it was no mistake, he did have terminal cancer. We wondered how much his autism was influencing his response to his illness, driving him to keep going.

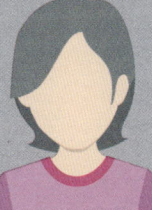
Marian
Mum

> These were experienced doctors and consultants who told us he only had a few months to live. No one expected him to live for nearly three years following his diagnosis and prognosis.

The care team had supported Stephane for many years and had a good understanding of what was important to him in his life and how his autism affected his thinking, social communication and relationships. However, our response to the diagnosis of a life-limiting illness is not something that any of us can easily predict. It was an area of support that the team had never before considered they would have to provide for Stephane, nor could they predict his response to his illness or what their roles would be in providing such support.

What is palliative care?

Palliative care is the care given to a person with an advanced, life-limiting illness which cannot be cured. It is about ensuring the best possible quality of life for that person during their illness from diagnosis through to the end of their life.

> *"Palliative care is an approach that improves the quality of life of patients and their families facing the problem(s) associated with life-threatening illness, through the prevention and relief of suffering by means of early identification and impeccable assessment and treatment of pain and other problems, physical, psychosocial and spiritual."*
>
> (World Health Organisation, 2015)

Palliative care isn't just about treating a person's medical and physical health needs. Understanding how to provide the best possible palliative and end of life care encompasses four key areas of support:

- **Physical** Supporting the person diagnosed with a life-limiting condition to cope with the physical implications of their illness. The person may require support to cope with distressing symptoms, get relief from pain and manage physical changes in themselves as a result of their illness. Physical care and support involves working very closely with healthcare professionals to ensure the individual is as comfortable and pain free as possible at the end of their life.

- **Psychological** Receiving a diagnosis of life-limiting illness is a psychologically challenging experience for the person diagnosed and for those closely involved in their life and care. The person diagnosed is likely to be coping with the loss of their emotional wellbeing as they try to come to terms with the implications of their illness and establish their wishes and aspirations for the end of their life.

- **Social** People diagnosed with a life-limiting illness are cited as vulnerable to loss of social relationships and networks as a result of the physical and psychological implications of their illness. It is important to consider how the person will maintain and in some cases redefine the relationships and interactions they have with the significant people within their life.

- **Spiritual** Spiritual themes and considerations often come to the fore in discussions about end of life care with an importance and immediacy unsurpassed by most other life events. Following a diagnosis of a life-limiting illness it is natural to consider themes such as personal meaning, culture, religion and self in the context of our own life and our relationship to the world around us.

When supporting people on the autism spectrum through palliative and end of life care it is important to consider how their autism will impact on each of these four key areas.

The issues explored when considering palliative and end of life care encompass many challenging, complex and important themes. Those diagnosed and the people close to them will face questions, decisions and experiences that we all would find difficult; these questions are often complicated by the challenges of the person's autism.

Pause for thought...

How will the person's differences in how they think and process information affect how we deliver care appropriate to their understanding, wishes and expectations?

How do we deliver appropriate care for individuals with social communication and interaction difficulties?

And how will sensory perceptual differences affect the individual's responses to illness, treatment or symptom control measures?

The autism spectrum

Providing end of life care to any person will always be a very individual process. It begins with an understanding of the person and what is important to them in life. However, for the team that supported Stephane it was important to stop and consider how the differing experiences and perceptions of someone on the autism spectrum might influence how they could deliver the best possible end of life care.

Autism is a lifelong, developmental condition that affects the way a person communicates, interacts with others and their environment, and processes information about the world around them. The autism spectrum refers to the range of ways the condition presents in an individual, which can vary greatly from person to person and throughout their life.

People on the autism spectrum are likely to have difficulty with **verbal and non-verbal communication**. Autism can affect a person's ability to understand, process and expressively use language and non-verbal means of communication.

People on the autism spectrum can have difficulty forming and sustaining **social relationships**. Their interactions with others may not appear typical and they may have difficulty understanding social rules and the intentions of others.

People on the autism spectrum are likely to have differing ways of **thinking, learning and processing information**. This can affect their ability to manage aspects of change and adapt to new and unfamiliar situations.

Sensory perceptual differences for people on the autism spectrum can affect the way they experience, interact with and process information about the world around them.

While some people on the autism spectrum will have subtle difficulties and live very independently, others will have more complex needs and require an intensive level of life-long support.

Scottish Autism have worked with an illustrator who has Asperger's Syndrome to create an interactive animated resource that demonstrates this.

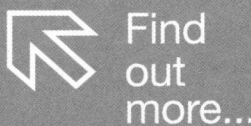

Find out more... www.understandingautism.org
This animated resource provides an accessible introduction to understanding the autism spectrum.

www.scottishautism.org

For the purposes of this practitioner resource we have focused on support for individuals on the autism spectrum who require a high level of support from families and care teams, and are therefore likely to have a learning disability.

However, some people without a learning disability may find that their viewpoint and perception of the world around them will be profoundly affected by their autism. It is worth remembering that the development of people on the autism spectrum is often uneven (Jordan, 2001), meaning that many individuals with autism will have areas of strength and ability as well as areas of complex difficulty. Describing individuals on the autism spectrum in terms such as 'high' or 'low' functioning can over-simplify and fail to appreciate the multi-faceted nature of how autism affects a person (Kenny et al, 2015).Therefore there may be information within this guide that is also relevant to more able individuals who face a specific support challenge as a result of their autism at the end of their life.

Despite growing interest in support for older people on the autism spectrum in recent years, there exists a lack of research and literature on the specific challenges of this type of support (Charlton and Happe, 2012) and also therefore on their palliative and end of life care needs. Much of the literature researched and referenced in the writing of this resource has been written specifically for the support of individuals with generic learning disabilities. Whilst people on the autism spectrum remain under-represented in the wider literature on palliative and end of life care, the literature reviewed for individuals with learning disabilities and communication difficulties will have clear links and relevance to the support needs of many people on the autism spectrum too.

People who experience barriers to engagement have a vulnerability in that their voice and experiences are not heard by health and social care services and decision makers (IRISS, 2010). It could be argued that there is a responsibility to consider how we share experiences and learning in an ethical way to support that dialogue between individuals, providers and policy makers. IRISS (Institute for Research and Innovation in Social Services) reflects on *"the role of personal storytelling in practice"*, advocating the value of this form of practice reflection, enriching understanding, engendering empathy, representing individual and shared realities and aiding learning and development (Drumm, 2013).

Predictably the complexities of Stephane's autism posed some unique challenges in providing palliative and end of life care to the team of people supporting him and they found it difficult to access information and resources that informed their practice. A 2010 article in the *Journal of Palliative Medicine* expressed concern that individual services within care organisations did not appear to share experiences of palliative care provision, resulting in a lack of wider sharing and learning (Ryan et al, 2010). This resource is our way of sharing a story, bringing together the key pieces of learning that informed our practice and reflecting on the things we have since discovered that we wish we had known.

Meet Stephane…

Having spent a long portion of his early years dividing his time between Scotland and France in the care of a loving and devoted family, Stephane came to live in supported accommodation with Scottish Autism when he was still a child. At the time of his diagnosis of terminal pancreatic cancer over 30 years later, he lived in a cluster of four flats surrounded by a peer group of fellow individuals on the autism spectrum whom he had known and grown up with throughout various life stages and transitions. He required 24-hour support to enable him to live as safely and independently as possible and support him to pursue meaningful life experiences based on what was important to him.

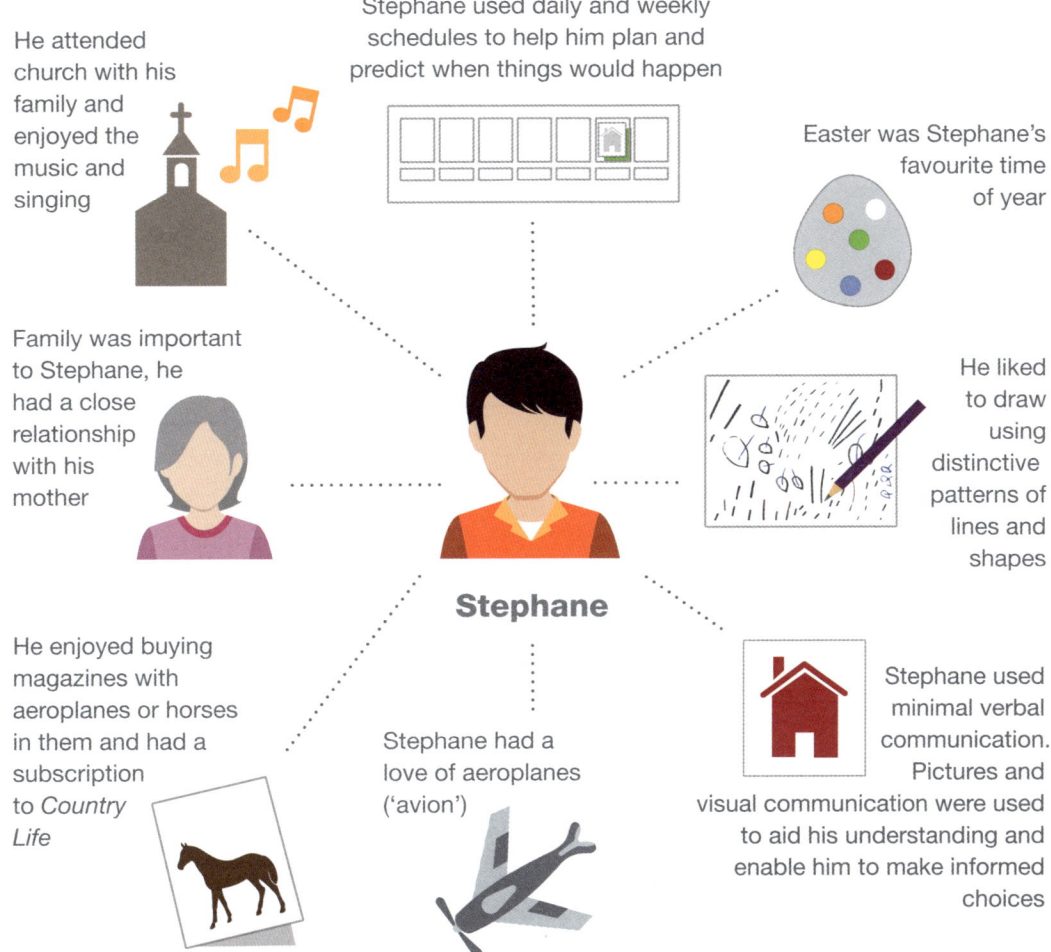

How Stephane's autism impacted on his life

Stephane was a 48 year old man with a diagnosis of autism and learning disabilities. While he was growing up in Scotland and France his family campaigned for greater understanding of the autism spectrum, at a time where there was far less autism awareness amongst professionals and the general public.

Stephane's expressive communication was affected by his autism and his use of conversational spoken word was limited. His verbal communication tended to be needs-led, or confined to use of particular key words and phrases. He would also communicate using echolalic repetition of words. This affected his ability to make informed choices and decisions in life as he would often repeat back the last choice offered or repeat the words of others. When stressed and anxious his words would become more clearly pronounced. Pictorial communication was routinely used to enable informed expression of choice and aid understanding.

Stephane had a good memory for events from his past as far back as his childhood, but had difficulty understanding the passing of time and required support with future planning. He used daily and weekly planners to reassure him and support his understanding of what would happen next. Sleep charts were used to count down to important events in his life.

Stephane was very motivated and driven by things that were of great importance to him. For other aspects of daily living he could be very passive and required promoting and support to motivate and engage him.

Familiarity helped Stephane find security and reassurance amongst the unpredictability of many aspects of life. Stephane was very routine driven and struggled with changes to things that were familiar to him. He liked to line up and order his belongings.

Stephane experienced sensory perceptual issues. He was sensitive to touch and disliked certain materials and textures touching his skin.

What was important in Stephane's life

Stephane had a passionate love of aeroplanes, inspired by his childhood and memories of his father. He loved to visit airports and transport museums and look at magazines about them. He was also fond of horses and cats and had a subscription to *Country Life* magazine.

Stephane had a unique style of drawing, creating rhythmic patterns of loops and lines inspired by the Aberdeen rain. He often used particular colours for certain days.

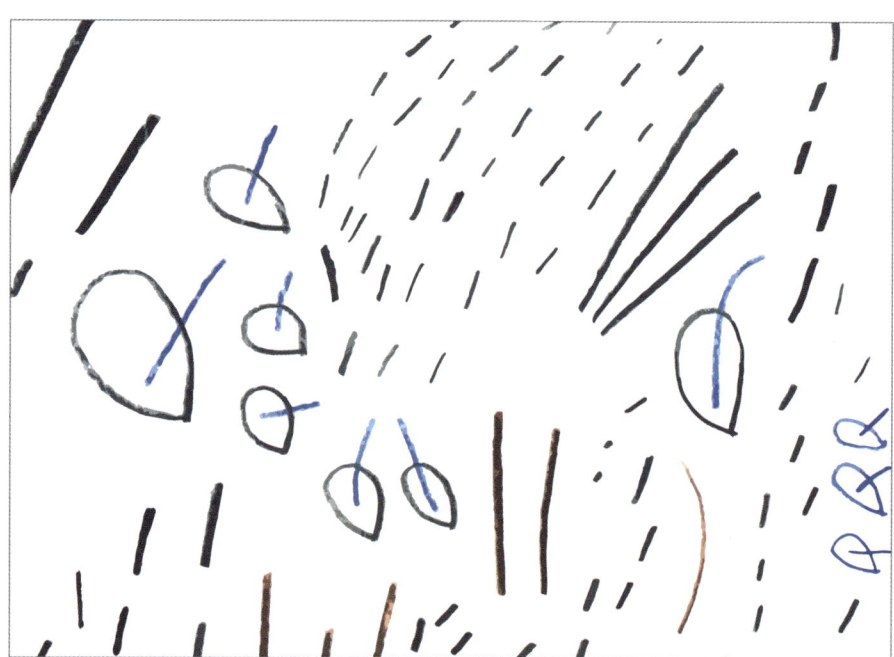

An example of Stephane's drawings

Stephane had a genuine love of all types of music. He was the first person out of the door at the prospect of an outing or venture, enjoying swimming, horse riding, walks on the beach and visits to structural landmarks such as bridges and castles.

Stephane was very motivated by his enjoyment of food and especially enjoyed eating out at Italian and Indian restaurants. Stephane enjoyed special occasions and Easter was his favourite time of year, motivated by a love of Easter eggs.

Relationships

Stephane liked people who were familiar and predictable in his life.

Stephane had difficulty initiating social contact and forming new relationships, but he had an extended group of friends and peers whom he had grown up with from childhood through to adulthood. He was an active participant in local day services and enjoyed social events and special occasions in the company of his support staff and friends.

Stephane had a very close relationship with his mother who was the most important person in his life. His brother and two sisters were very close to him growing up and his mother recalls Stephane's love and affection for them. His mother lived in Aberdeen but would travel down often and had a very active part in both Stephane's life and the wider Scottish Autism community. Stephane's father passed away when he was ten years old. Stephane attended his funeral and would point to the sky to gesture that his father was in heaven now. Stephane's father was French and there were both French and Scottish influences in family life as he was growing up. Stephane attended church with his family and enjoyed the music and singing within the church, with Amazing Grace a remembered favourite.

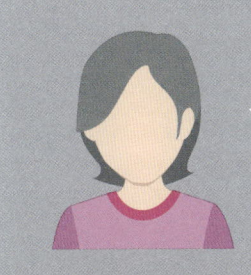

Stephane was a very sensitive person. He loved aeroplanes and as a child was often on an aeroplane coming back to Aberdeen from France. He loved 'avion, avion, avion!'

Marian
Mum

Meet the team…

Following Stephane's death the team who supported him at the end of his life had opportunities to discuss how they felt, reflect on what they personally found difficult, what the team did well and what we could learn from to inform our practice for the future. These conversations were filmed and transcribed and this has formed the basis of the work done in compiling this resource.

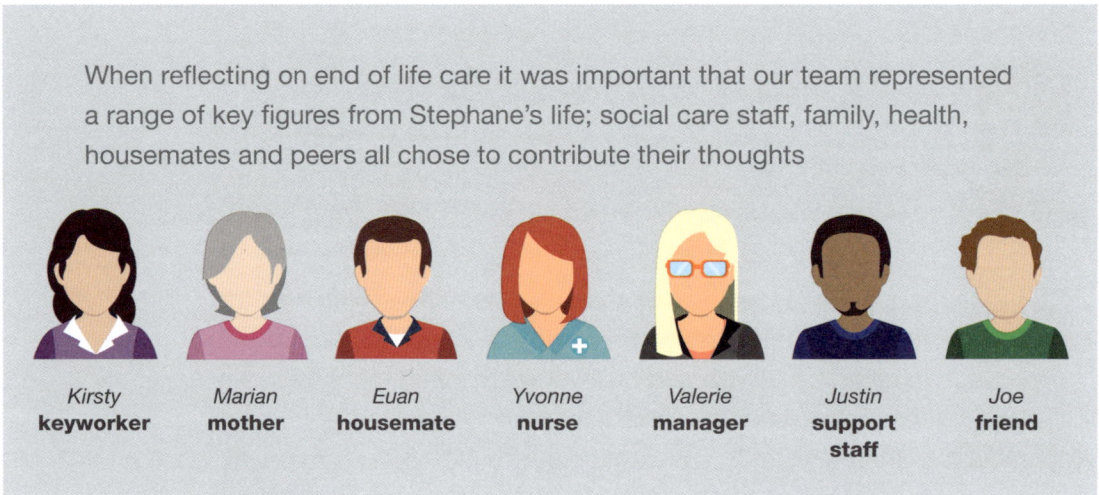

When reflecting on end of life care it was important that our team represented a range of key figures from Stephane's life; social care staff, family, health, housemates and peers all chose to contribute their thoughts

Kirsty **keyworker** — *Marian* **mother** — *Euan* **housemate** — *Yvonne* **nurse** — *Valerie* **manager** — *Justin* **support staff** — *Joe* **friend**

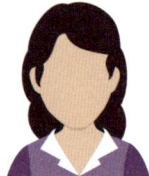

Kirsty is a practitioner from the Scottish Autism care team that provided direct care and support to Stephane in his home. Kirsty was Stephane's **keyworker** at the time of his diagnosis through to the end of his life. The team were continually engaged in reviewing Stephane's changing care needs and establishing the wishes and aspirations of Stephane and his family as he approached the end of his life.

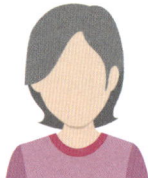

Marian was Stephane's **mother** and represents his family in our reflections on his end of life care. Stephane's father had passed away when he was young, and his mother was the most important person in his life. Marian was very supportive of Stephane's care team.

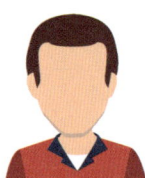

Euan was Stephane's **housemate** and lived with him in a supported accommodation flat with 24-hour support from Scottish Autism. Euan is also on the autism spectrum, and had known and lived with Stephane for many years.

Peaceful, Pain Free and Dignified

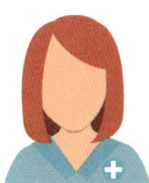
Yvonne was Stephane's **community palliative care nurse**. She provided hands-on nursing care, and advised on pain and symptom control. Yvonne was also an excellent support to Stephane's staff team, providing them with invaluable practical and emotional support.

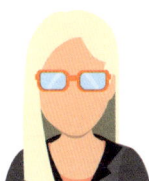
Valerie is the **manager** of the Scottish Autism care team that supported Stephane within his home. Valerie was responsible for leading the team of autism support staff that cared for Stephane at the time of his diagnosis through to the end of his life.

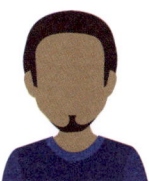
Justin is a representative from the Scottish Autism **support worker** team that supported Stephane in 24-hour care. Stephane's team comprised of a core team of six support workers who had all worked with and known him prior to his diagnosis. The same support team continued to support him through to the end of his life.

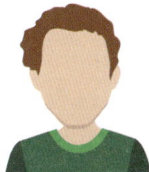
Joe was a **friend** and peer of Stephane's who had known him since childhood. Joe is also on the autism spectrum and attended the same day service as Stephane.

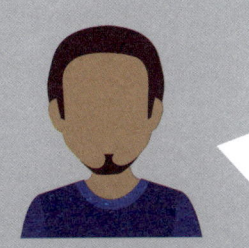
Justin
Support worker

> We were all in this together, we were all in this for Stephane. The way the team worked together to support him was amazing. Many of us had never gone through this, even with a family member. Everyone involved in his care had exactly the same priorities, to make Stephane comfortable and happy as best we could.

> The key for me was close working between the autism support staff and the community team; with consultants, GP, district nurses, social workers all making sure that everything was going to run smoothly.

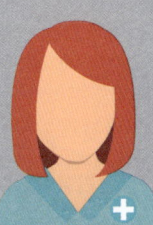
Yvonne
Nurse

Many practitioners working with people on the autism spectrum will never have supported a person through palliative and end of life care. However, as we support people with autism through their whole life journey we will be increasingly faced with issues of illness, palliative and end of life care.

In her 2001 publication *Support for the Bereaved and Dying in Services for Adults with Autism Spectrum Disorders*, Helen Green Allison identifies the importance of good relationships between the three key groups involved in palliative care of the dying: the care staff, the healthcare professionals and the family of the patient. Specific advice for working together effectively includes:

- Invite key health contacts to join team meetings
- Establish communication protocols for sharing information between health and social care teams and family members
- Don't be afraid to ask questions!

In addition to the key groups noted above there may be a range of people and professionals involved in the person's care at the end of their life, each with their own area of specialism or knowledge. Best practice in palliative care recognises the value of effective multiagency working to ensure the best possible quality of support for the person diagnosed with a terminal illness.

GP	Therapeutic practitioners	Family	Department for Work and Pensions (DWP)
Consultant	Counselling services and support groups	Next of kin	Funding/local authority
District nurse	Advice and information services	Befriender	Attorney
Specialist nurses	Specialist training providers	Friends	Solicitor
Palliative care team	Social care staff	Peer group	Mental Welfare Commission
Occupational therapist	Autism support team	Housemate	Advocacy services
Psychologist	Social work	Church Synagogue Mosque	
Speech and language		Religious and spiritual figures	
Community learning disability services			

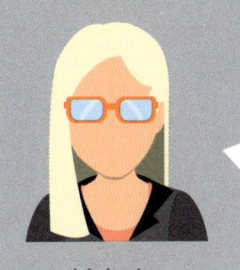

> We couldn't have done it without everyone working together as a team, and it really did show the importance of a multi-disciplinary approach. Working together with the family and the healthcare team to be the best we could be for Stephane.

Valerie
Manager

This resource has been written for fellow social care practitioners, based on our experiences and discussions with colleagues, families and professionals. No one can claim to have all the answers about supporting someone on the autism spectrum through what will always be a very personal and individual experience. Those supporting that person must sensitively try to capture a holistic picture of what is important to that person, both throughout their life and at the end of their life. It is about enabling them to have the best possible quality of life in the time that the individual has left as well as preparing for death. And as the end of life approaches, we are trying to achieve:

> *"a good death; peaceful, pain free and dignified."*
>
> (Yvonne, Community palliative care nurse)

Chapter 1:
Physical

Palliative and end of life care inevitably involves supporting the person diagnosed with a life-limiting condition to cope with the physical implications of their illness. The person may require support to cope with distressing symptoms, get relief from pain and manage physical changes in themselves as a result of their illness. It involves working very closely with healthcare professionals to ensure the individual is as comfortable and pain free as possible at the end of their life.

Stephane's story

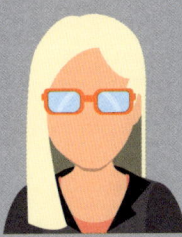

Valerie
Manager

When staff started to spot that there was something not quite right with Stephane's health, he had lost weight and was more tired than usual. We felt there was a change and we wanted it investigated further. We had several appointments with GPs to request a referral to a consultant. When we finally got an appointment they were reluctant to give him a scan, as they thought it was his diabetes and change of diet. Stephane wasn't able to use his voice in these appointments, so we had to really keep pushing to say we wanted the scan. And when he did get the scan and the results came back they sent them back to another specialist to take another look. They were shocked by what they had found, and called us back in to tell us that with the size of the tumour they had found in Stephane's pancreas he would have three to six months to live. They had never seen someone with a tumour the size that Stephane had display loss of weight and tiredness as the only symptoms of such an advanced illness.

There are often challenges in effectively managing the healthcare needs of individuals on the autism spectrum and those with learning disabilities, and many reasons why they might not present typically or be able to communicate or engage in consultation and treatment with healthcare professionals.

> *"The main obstacle in medical assessment is found to be communication problems. Other barriers include a lack of understanding of health matters and difficulties in following medical instructions, lack of medical notes and history due to previously fragmented care."*
>
> (Tuffrey-Wijne, 2003)

Pause for thought...

What implications does this have for diagnosis of serious illness and appropriate treatment plans for individuals on the autism spectrum with an advanced or life-limiting illness?

We asked support staff working in autism services what some of the challenges were in managing the physical healthcare needs of the individuals on the autism spectrum they know and support. The challenges most commonly cited were:

- lack of obvious or typical presentation of symptoms
- non-typical reaction to and expression of pain
- sensory perceptual differences and difficulties
- lack of awareness or understanding of own body
- lack of understanding/appropriate education about the implications and consequences of health problems
- unclear expectations about what will happen and how it will feel
- communication barriers, potentially leading to missed or misdiagnosis
- the requirement to follow social cues and rules in a healthcare setting
- issues with capacity and consent to treatment
- resistance to engaging with health services due to heightened stress and anxieties
- the impact of negative past experiences on future confidence
- lack of awareness in others of how the person's autism may present barriers to best possible healthcare and willingness of others to make accommodations based on that

The Department of Health's *Confidential Inquiry into the Deaths of People with Learning Disabilities* (Heslop et al, 2013) recognises the extreme vulnerability of individuals with learning disabilities including those on the autism spectrum and made the following recommendation to healthcare providers:

> *"Recommendation 7: People with learning disabilities to have access to the same investigations and treatments as anyone else, but acknowledging and accommodating that they may need to be delivered differently to achieve the same outcome.*
>
> *Given the problems that people with learning disabilities experience with having their illness diagnosed we recommend that investigations be undertaken early in the care pathways of people with learning disabilities. This is a recommendation for all healthcare providers."*
>
> (Heslop et al, 2013)

Good relationships based on mutual understanding between people on the autism spectrum and healthcare professionals are essential to ensure appropriate diagnosis and treatment planning. This involves recognition on the part of healthcare professionals that accommodations may have to be made to enable someone to access essential healthcare as is their right.

Where there are barriers to that dialogue between individuals on the autism spectrum and healthcare professionals it is essential that families and social care staff advocate on behalf of the person and work in partnership with health colleagues to ensure best possible care for the person they are supporting.

For individuals who struggle to effectively communicate their needs with healthcare professionals, healthcare and communication passports can provide valuable and important information to ensure best possible person centred care and treatment. Use of such passports can support healthcare staff in understanding how the person's autism will affect their ability to cope with consultations, investigations and medical treatment. They will also provide important information about the person's healthcare needs and medical history.

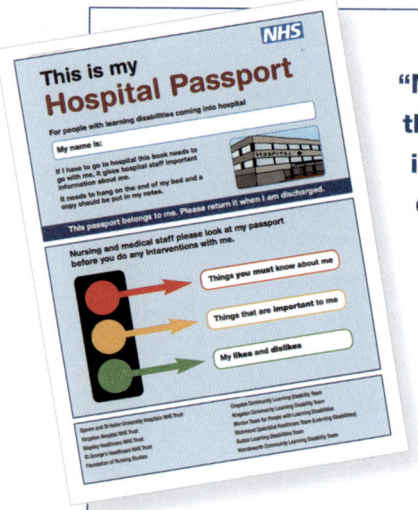

"Many families and paid carers report the difficulties they face in getting health professionals to take crucial information about the needs of the person with a learning disability into account. Rather than seeing attempts to share such knowledge as a hindrance, professionals should use it to help them meet the needs of their patients. There are now excellent tools to assist in passing over this essential information, such as hospital passports, grab sheets and communication books."

(Mencap, 2007)

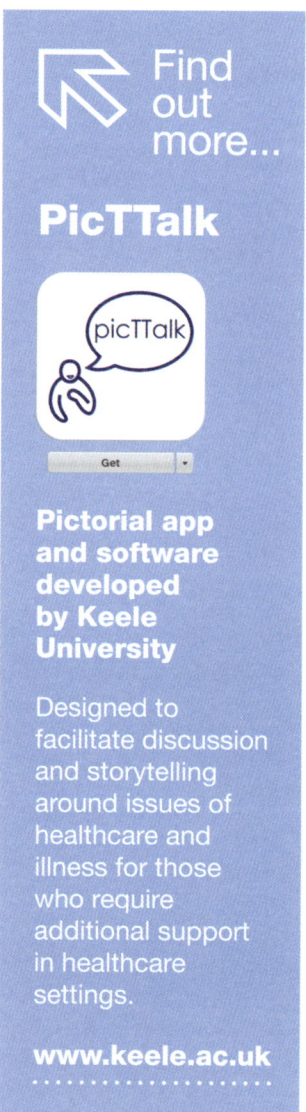

Your local NHS trust should be able to provide you with a locally used version of a hospital passport to aid important sharing of knowledge that informs the individual's care in a hospital setting.

Other resources and applications to facilitate discussion and patient centred care are available. PicTTalk is an example of a simple pictorial app designed to facilitate discussion between professionals and patients with autism and/or learning disabilities around their care and treatment. In addition to more general medical images it contains a mode specifically for discussion about sensitive issues of death and dying.

Health services are legally required to make *reasonable adjustments* for individuals on the autism spectrum under the Equality Act (2010), to ensure fair and equitable treatment. When looking specifically at palliative and end of life care, this not only has implications for early diagnosis and treatment of potentially life-limiting illnesses, but also for the process of appropriate care planning following diagnosis of an incurable, advanced and life-limiting condition.

Care planning

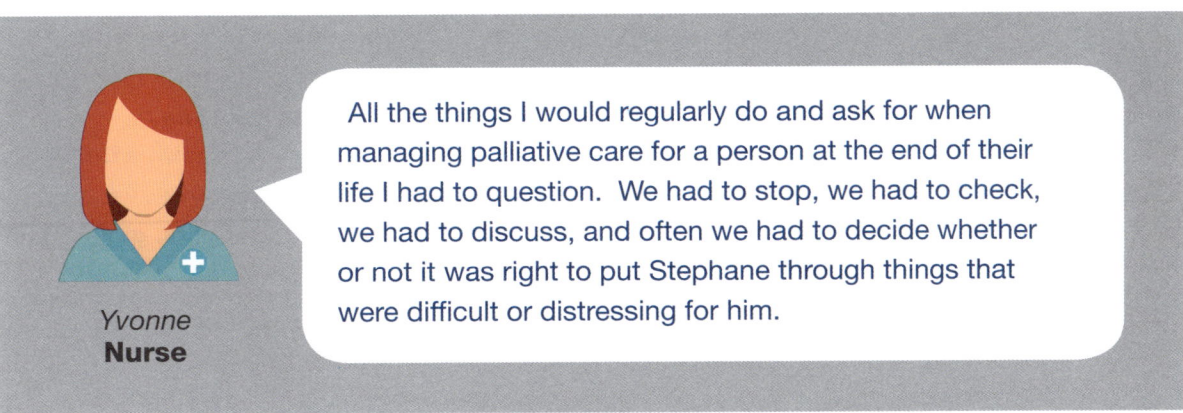

Yvonne **Nurse**

"All the things I would regularly do and ask for when managing palliative care for a person at the end of their life I had to question. We had to stop, we had to check, we had to discuss, and often we had to decide whether or not it was right to put Stephane through things that were difficult or distressing for him."

Some of the particular challenges raised by the palliative care nurses in managing Stephane's end of life treatment were:

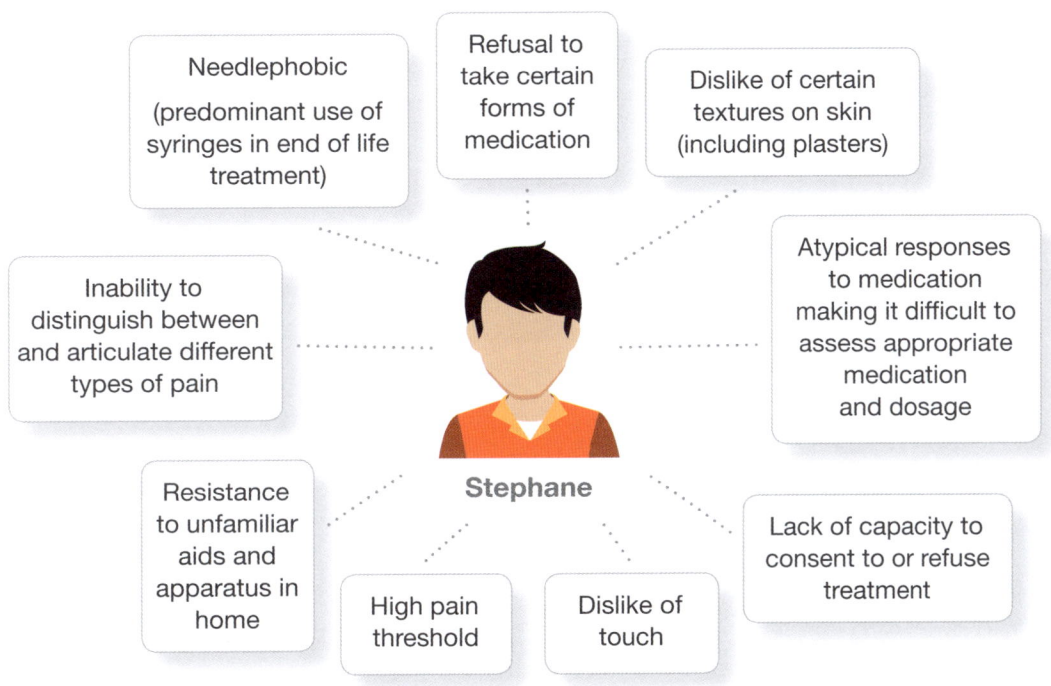

- Needlephobic (predominant use of syringes in end of life treatment)
- Refusal to take certain forms of medication
- Dislike of certain textures on skin (including plasters)
- Atypical responses to medication making it difficult to assess appropriate medication and dosage
- Inability to distinguish between and articulate different types of pain
- Resistance to unfamiliar aids and apparatus in home
- High pain threshold
- Dislike of touch
- Lack of capacity to consent to or refuse treatment

"Practitioners in both acute and primary health care services need to appreciate the myriad ways in which treatment can be compromised by an autism spectrum condition, as failure to comply is an oft-quoted reason why the health outcomes of people with autism may be perceived as less successful than for the 'neurotypical' patient."

(Morton-Cooper, 2004)

Each person on the autism spectrum will have their own challenges to overcome when engaging in consultations, medical procedures and the level of physical and medical care required in palliative and end of life care. An enabling person centred approach should be taken to support people on the autism spectrum to overcome those challenges, and accommodations made where possible that recognise the diversity of needs in the patient group.

Mencap's report *Death by Indifference* (2007) expresses concern that healthcare professionals can make assumptions about an individual's ability to tolerate procedures and treatment. They recommend that:

> *"As with any patient, treatment and interventions for someone with a learning disability should be considered on a case by case basis and, where reasonable adjustments are given proper consideration and planning, most treatments can be administered."*

Following the publication of *Death by Indifference*, Mencap launched their Getting it Right Charter in 2010. It provides health trusts and organisations with guidance on how they can improve the healthcare of people with learning disabilities. Recommendations include ensuring that information is available in accessible formats, routine use of hospital passports and the appointment of learning disability liaison nurses in hospitals.

Many people on the autism spectrum struggle to access healthcare facilities and hospitals and may require accommodations to be made to help them do so. Your local health authority may employ someone whose role it is to enable such accommodations to be made, such as a designated learning disability liaison nurse. Community learning disability nurses may also be available to provide support to care teams and bridge a gap between health and social care, or your local NHS may be able to identify a nominated link worker who can support staff training and understanding across areas of specialism (Cross et al, 2012). You can contact your regional NHS board to find out what support is available in your local area.

Pain management and medication

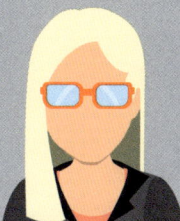
Valerie **Manager**

Stephane's autism definitely seemed to impact on his pain threshold. Stephane appeared to be able to manage and handle a lot more pain than a typical individual. This was difficult for GPs and nurses to understand because they also had never dealt with an individual with autism who presented like Stephane at this stage of his life, and care staff who knew him had to push to say these are very subtle signs but we know he's uncomfortable.

Stephane's tolerance of medications and his inability to distinguish between different types of pain made it difficult to manage his pain relief at the end of his life. The doses of drugs we were using were very, very high. We had to think about side effects and how we would identify them, such as hallucination, or if he became toxic on his medication. That was a fear of mine. The resistance his body had to medication that had been built up over many years, in addition to dealing with usual end of life medical management, made the whole end of life care that bit more challenging for me. But I'm glad because that's how I learn and I hope I can bring that experience forward for another person.

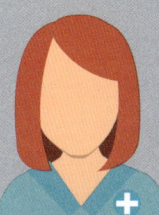
Yvonne **Nurse**

"Every member of staff whose role involves pain treatment needs to be aware of the potential difficulties in diagnosing pain... This is especially important in cases that involve people with limited verbal communication. Staff must be trained to overcome issues around communication in order to bring about the best outcome for the patient."

(Mencap, 2007)

Pain assessment tools use a range of vocabulary to describe pain to support appropriate and effective pain management.

"Tender, crushing, squeezing, stabbing, sharp, electric shock, aching, sore, burning, continuous, intermittent, occasional, throbbing, dull, discomfort."

(Supportive Care Register, 2014)

Pause for thought...

How do the individuals on the autism spectrum you know and support express pain and discomfort?

Chapter 1: **Physical**

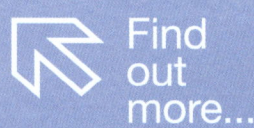

Find out more...

DisDAT

Disability Distress Assessment Tool

The DisDAT tool is designed to help identify distress cues in individuals who have complex communication challenges.

It can be used by support teams to document indicators of distress or discomfort and inform clinical decisions regarding the person's care.

www.disdat.co.uk

For individuals on the autism spectrum who experience issues with sensory perceptual differences or social communication, it can be difficult to articulate and express pain and discomfort in a typical way. Management of pain in end of life care is dependent on the person being able to communicate how they feel, to be descriptive of pain and what they are feeling at a level of sensation.

In her publication *Health Care and the Autism Spectrum*, Alison Morton-Cooper highlights the lack of studies into pain management for people on the autism spectrum but acknowledges *"the possibility that standard pharmacological responses to pain may be insufficient to the task of relieving pain in individuals with autism"*. This makes it all the more vital that there is a detailed history available of how a person has previously responded to medical interventions to ensure clinically effective treatment (Morton-Cooper, 2004).

It is therefore important that care staff and anyone required to advocate on behalf of that person are clear about how the person with autism expresses pain and discomfort to ensure appropriate management of symptoms.

> *"It is important to remember that patients with limited or no communication still experience pain even though they cannot report it. Observation of behaviour and physical signs that may be associated with pain will provide additional information but correlation between observer- and patient-reported pain may be poor."*
>
> (Faull et al, 2012)

It may be useful to look at tools such as the DisDAT Disability Distress Assessment Tool (Regnard et al, 2006) to identify indicators of pain in the person with autism you support if they have complex communication challenges that leave them vulnerable to poor assessment of pain levels.

Scales for expressing pain

Making an individual comfortable and pain free at the end of their life is the key priority for all those involved in that person's care. If the person with autism is unable to typically express or articulate their level of pain or discomfort then there are pain assessment tools that make use of visual and written scales of pain ranging from mild to severe.

For example:

- The Wong-Baker FACES ® pain rating scale is a pictorial way of communicating pain levels. The visual nature of it will work well for some people on the autism spectrum, particularly if they have previously been taught to label how they feel in a similar way. However, it is dependent on the patient's ability to read and understand symbols representing facial expressions and to relate that to their physical and emotional states, which may be very difficult for other individuals.

- The Abbey Pain Scale (Abbey et al, 1998-2002) is a pain assessment tool for patients with communication difficulties, rating pain levels based on observations relating to vocalisations, expression, behavioural and physiological changes in a person's presentation.

The Scottish Government's *The Keys to Life* strategy recognises that individuals with learning disabilities may be at higher risk of physical or mental ill health and consequently may be prescribed multiple drugs with the potential to adversely affect health through side effects and drug interactions (Scottish Government, 2013). It follows this is then likely to be true for many of the individuals with a diagnosis of autism who are under the health care of local learning disability or mental health teams. There exists a broad variability in how people respond to prescribed drugs across the general population (Twycross et al, 2015). Some individuals on the autism spectrum may have a specific response to medication and/or their previous medical history may affect how they respond to the drugs prescribed for symptom control during end of life care.

This may affect the drugs and dosage of medication prescribed by health professionals.

Controlled Drugs are prescribed medications that are usually used to treat severe pain or induce anaesthesia. There are additional safety precautions and requirements around their administration and storage that social care services must adhere to. These additional measures include requirements around prescription, administration, records, storage and disposal of such medication.

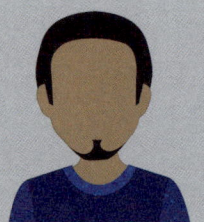

Justin
Support worker

There were a lot of controlled drugs coming in and out of Stephane's home at the time and the regulations around their storage and administration were different from those that we were used to managing.

I did check with the GP about how we stored and managed the medication and we were initially told that our existing systems would be adequate even though it transpired there were additional measures we required to put in place. But I contacted the Care Inspectorate pharmacist and they were really helpful and advised us on how to store the medication.

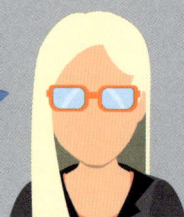

Valerie
Manager

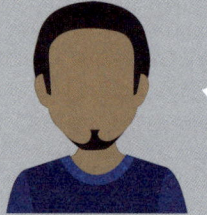

Justin
Support worker

It was important that everyone in the support team knew what the drugs were and what they were used for. And because there were often changes we needed to have tight controls and clear communication between all members of the team to make sure important information was passed on correctly and accurately.

Anticipatory drugs are medications prescribed in advance of their use for pain management and symptom control by the person's GP or palliative care specialist. This ensures they are quickly available to help with anticipated acute episodes of pain and distressing symptoms. The medication and any associated apparatus for administration should be available in the patient's home so they are available for the attending clinician. They should be stored as per other controlled drugs in what is often referred to as a *"just in case box"* (British Medical Association, 2015).

Medication will often be delivered through use of a syringe driver in the latter stages of a person's palliative care. A syringe driver is a portable pump that will be set up by a nurse or doctor to deliver a continuous dose of a drug from a syringe through a small needle inserted under the skin of the arm or abdomen.

For information and advice on **handling medication** see the Royal Pharmaceutical Society's *The Handling of Medicines in Social Care*, which provides guidance on the handling of medicines that complies with best practice guidance, National Care Standards, and relevant legislation (www.rpharms.com).

For guidance and legislation specific to the use of controlled drugs, see:

- *A Guide to Good Practice in the Management of Controlled Drugs in Primary Care* – Scotland 2012
- *Safer Management of Controlled Drugs: A guide to good practice in primary care* (Northern Ireland)
- *Safer Management of Controlled Drugs: A guide to good practice in primary care* (England)

Where a person has died in supported care, registered managers and staff teams must ensure that all medication is kept for at least seven days before being returned to a pharmacist for disposal. Medication may be requested as evidence where there is the need for a coroner's inquest into the person's death (Regulation and Quality Improvement Authority, 2011).

Managing symptoms and the effects of illness

Social care staff are unlikely to have a developed understanding of what symptoms, presentations and secondary complications are likely to arise when supporting someone on the autism spectrum following a diagnosis of life-limiting illness. It is essential they have opportunities to ask questions and are informed of what measures they can take to help the person they are supporting feel as comfortable as possible as their illness progresses.

Some of the issues that typically need to be addressed for people with a life-limiting illness might include:

- mouth care to prevent dehydration
- skin care to avoid sores
- continence care/support
- weight loss
- sleep issues
- tiredness and fatigue
- sickness and nausea

- eating difficulties and loss of appetite
- breathlessness
- fluid build-up
- risk of infection
- side effects of medications

Support is available from a range of individuals in primary health care teams, in addition to the palliative care nurses, to support with symptom management (for example, district nurses, dieticians and physiotherapists). Complementary therapists may also be able to support with alleviation of symptoms and promoting physical wellbeing.

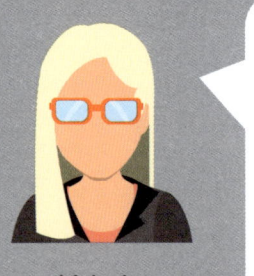

Valerie
Manager

> The nurses gave us so many tips and suggestions for keeping Stephane comfortable, they were a great source of advice. They gave us simple suggestions such as using fans to reduce sweating, and ice and frozen fruit to prevent dehydration of the mouth. They let us know what to look out for when using care aids such as catheters and talked through some of the symptoms we could expect to see as Stephane's health deteriorated.
>
> My advice to care teams would be don't ever be afraid to ask. It is normal to feel that this type of care is out of your comfort zone or beyond your knowledge. We had the nurses on speed dial and they came along to our team meetings so we had plenty of opportunities to ask questions.

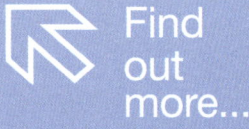 Find out more...

End of Life: a guide

A booklet for people in the final stages of life and their carers

This booklet jointly produced by Marie Curie and Macmillan contains information about what to expect in the way of physical changes and symptoms as someone approaches the end of their life.

www.mariecurie.org.uk

Peaceful, Pain Free and Dignified

Advance care planning

Advance care planning (ACP) encourages discussion between the person with a life-limiting illness and their health and care providers. The aim of ACP is to enable the individual to communicate their wishes for their care prior to a significant deterioration in their health that may result in diminished capacity or ability to communicate their wishes.

NHS England's *Deciding Right* is an initiative in north-east England concerned with promoting best practice in advanced care decisions. The *Deciding Right* strategy expresses concern about *"poor or absent dialogue between the individuals and healthcare professionals resulting in a lack of shared decision making"* (Regnard, 2014).

Advance decisions to refuse treatment (ADRTs) are legally binding agreements where an individual refuses to consent to specific treatments in advance of loss of capacity. Where an individual has capacity at the time of making the decision they may choose to refuse particular forms of life-sustaining treatment in the advanced stages of their illness. A patient cannot refuse basic care that is about keeping them comfortable. An ADRT ensures that their views are understood and respected ahead of any loss of capacity as a result of their illness. In England and Wales this process can only be done in compliance with the Mental Capacity Act (2005) and is guided by the MCA Codes of Practice. In Scotland and Northern Ireland an advance decision is also legally binding but governed by common law instead of an act.

Deciding Right (Regnard, 2014) details the guiding principles behind ADRTs. Guidance is also available online from the Macmillan website www.macmillan.org.uk.

Assessment of capacity should be done in accordance with the Mental Capacity Act or Adults with Incapacity (Scotland) Act. This states that all adults have the right to make their own decisions, or be given as much help as possible to do so before being determined as unable to make decisions.

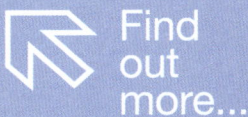

Find out more...

Deciding Right

NHS Northern England Strategic Clinical Networks

The *Deciding Right* decision aid and app for smartphone are available to help guide individuals and carers through the process of making advance care decisions. It is designed to promote choice and empowerment, particularly for those who are deemed to lack capacity to self advocate or engage in complex decisions affecting their care.

www.nescn.
nhs.uk/
deciding-right

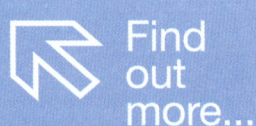

Find out more...

Advance Care Planning: A guide for health and social care staff

NHS's *Advance Care Planning Guide* contains information on advance care planning, defining capacity and professional responsibilities relating to ACP.

www.endoflife careforadults .nhs.uk

A person is defined as lacking capacity to make a decision if they cannot:

- understand the information relevant to the decision
- retain that information
- use or weigh that information as part of the decision-making process
- communicate that decision.

If an individual lacks capacity to make decisions regarding their care and treatment then family and carers may not automatically have the right to make decisions for them. Decisions may fall to the lead healthcare practitioner.

A **power of attorney** may be appointed to make decisions based on the best interests of the person if they are deemed not to have capacity. This person can also be named in advance if the person is at risk of losing capacity due to the nature of their life-limiting illness. (See the Mental Capacity Act (2005), Adults with Incapacity (Scotland) Act (2000) and MCA Codes of Practice for health and social care professionals.)

If an individual does not have the capacity to enter into a process of advance care planning every effort should still be made to determine their wishes. Whilst not legally binding, this can be documented in the form of a statement of wishes and preferences which can still be used to inform care and treatment.

For people on the autism spectrum who have differing communication preferences and ways of processing information, changes to how we present information and choices to them can have a significant effect on their capacity to make decisions about their care. The British Institute of Learning Disabilities recognises that individuals with complex communication challenges are in danger of being excluded from decisions that affect their lives unless those around them are prepared to change (Jones, 2002). It is always important to consider: does the person lack capacity to make a decision about their care, or have we failed to make changes and put in the correct supports to enable them to understand their choices and make informed decisions?

Do not attempt cardiopulmonary resuscitation orders

A **do not attempt cardiopulmonary resuscitation order** (DNACPR) is a decision to no longer attempt cardiopulmonary resuscitation. It applies only to CPR and does not imply that any other form of treatment will be withdrawn or withheld (General Medical Council, 2010). It is a decision that can be taken by lead healthcare clinicians if deemed clinically appropriate and is based on a full and considered evaluation of an individual's case.

In non-emergency situations DNACPRs should always be discussed with individuals and their families.

There has been concern expressed about the potential for poor adherence to DNACPR guidelines for people with learning disabilities and those who struggle to have a voice in decisions affecting their care and treatment (Heslop et al, 2013). In 2012 an NHS hospital in Kent was sued following the issuing of a DNACPR order by the doctor on duty, citing the man's learning difficulties amongst their reasons for no resuscitation (Meikle, 2012). The individual's family and carers were not aware of the order until it was discovered on his discharge; they had a very different assessment of his quality of life than the lead clinician who had issued the order.

The Scottish Government published a policy on DNACPR in 2010 that states:

> *"Quality of life judgements should not be part of the decision-making process for healthcare professionals.*
>
> *This policy adopts the view that clinical decisions should be based on immediate health needs and not on a professional's opinion on quality of life. This is primarily because opinions on quality of life made by health professionals are very subjective and often at variance with the views of the patient and relevant others."*

(Scottish Government, 2010)

Discriminatory circumstances such as the case cited are extreme, but are worth reflecting on when supporting a person who is potentially subject to the judgements of someone in a clinical setting who does not have a developed and holistic understanding of the person and their life. Individuals with communication and capacity challenges who are at the end of their life may be dependent on family, advocates and people of trust to liaise with lead healthcare professionals to inform aspects of decision making in such important circumstances.

> **Pause for thought…**
>
> Whoever is deemed to have the decision-making responsibilities, it is essential that the wishes of the person are heard and at the centre of all decision making processes.

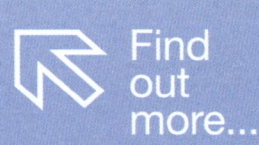

Find out more...

Living and Dying Well: A national action plan for palliative and end of life care in Scotland

A framework for delivering person centred services for individuals requiring palliative and end of life care in Scotland.

www.scotland.gov.uk

Electronic palliative care summary/co-ordination systems

An **electronic palliative care summary** (ePCS) or **electronic palliative care coordination system** (EPaCCS) can be kept by healthcare professionals involved in the individual's care with consent from the individual and their carers. EPaCCS are designed to ensure effective and responsive sharing of important information regarding an individual's care preferences.

Where an ePCS is in use, twice daily information regarding the person's palliative care needs is updated on an electronic database from the patient's GP records and made accessible to out-of-hours services, accident and emergency and ambulance services and NHS 24. This is designed to enable appropriate sharing of important information regarding the individual's treatment and care.

For more information on ePCS see NHS Scotland's *Living and Dying Well: A national action plan for palliative and end of life care in Scotland*.

Support environments

Home or hospice

When someone is diagnosed with a terminal or life-limiting illness they may not be well enough to remain within their own home when their physical health deteriorates. The requirement for specialist nursing care may mean that in the latter stages of their illness they need to stay in a hospital or hospice where there are staff who can address the complexities of their healthcare needs. However, there are also many individuals who choose to remain within their own home and for people on the autism spectrum who struggle with change and transition the move to an unfamiliar environment may be particularly difficult to cope with in addition to the stresses of their illness and prognosis.

Accounts from individuals going through palliative care describe how their anxieties about moving to a hospice were alleviated once they had visited the hospice and realised it was a safe space. They felt they then had clearer expectations of the environment because they had been "*put fully in the picture*" (Beresford et al, 2006). This may be especially true for individuals on the autism spectrum whose issues with predictive and flexible thinking may mean that they need support to more fully imagine what moving to a hospice involves. Visits to support environments and use of pictorial or video supports may help a person on the autism spectrum make a more informed decision about hospice care. In the event that decision is taken out of their hands it might also help to have done preparatory work that makes such a big transition less frightening for someone with unclear expectations about what hospice care involves.

Social Stories™ can be used to help an individual on the autism spectrum anticipate what to expect in a particular situation. They could be a useful way to explore and explain some of the anticipated treatments and experiences a person on the autism spectrum may have trouble envisioning. This can be useful for those individuals who don't understand treatment plans or the terminology typically used. Also, for individuals who have trouble around future planning, this can be a useful way to firm up expectations. This has to be done sensitively and support teams may feel they require the support of a speech and language therapist and/or their local learning disability team for advice and support.

Communication formats such as photographs, symbols, help cards and body charts were all used to support Stephane's understanding of what to expect in the way of care and treatment. They were also used to enable him to express his own experiences of pain and discomfort and to ask for help when he needed support to manage the symptoms of his ill health.

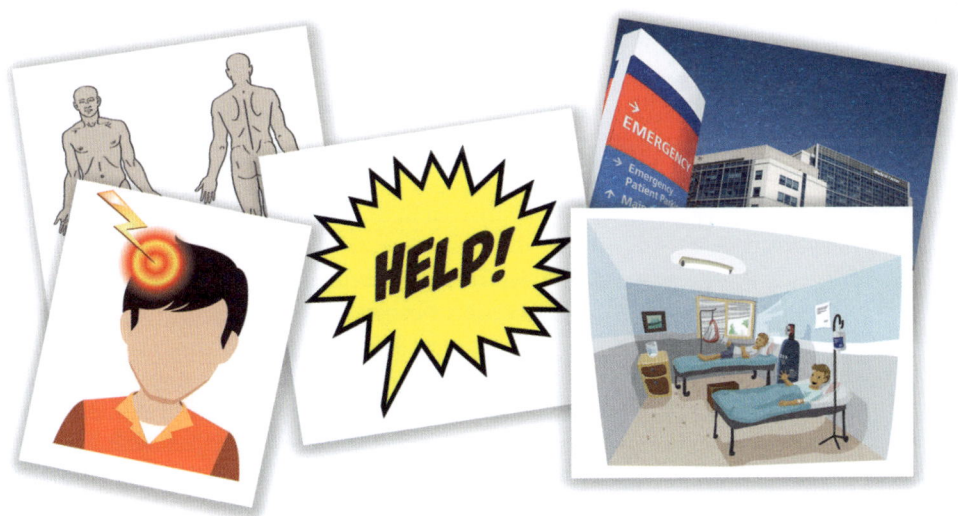

If a person chooses to remain in their own home then they will have the support of their local GP, community nurses and palliative care teams. The GP will take the lead in coordinating their patient's care and making the necessary referrals to primary healthcare teams.

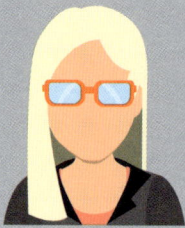

Valerie
Manager

This was outwith our remit, our knowledge. So we spoke to the local hospice and the family and we decided it would be best for Stephane to try and remain in his home. We did discuss shared care with the hospice in the event that he could no longer stay in his home, with his autism support staff going into the hospice and supporting the nursing staff to understand the impact of his autism on his care needs. Fortunately he was able to stay in his home until he passed away. But the point at which we crossed the line into nursing care and the role we had as support staff was hard to define, and we didn't realise how much nursing care was going to be involved in his support.

The health team thought, 'How are we going to do this? How will the care team manage this?' It was very much like I was having to do informal education with the care staff all the time as we went through the process. I remember thinking this must be overwhelming for this team because they've never been in a scenario like this, but they were learning and listening and taking it all in.

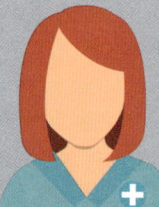

Yvonne
Nurse

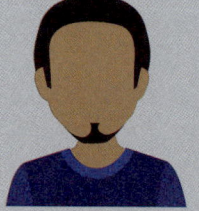

Justin
Support worker

It was complex because we were social care staff but at the time it felt like nursing too. Things I thought I'd never be able to do just became everyday routine.

Peaceful, Pain Free and Dignified

If the person with a life-limiting illness needs to move from their home to a hospice or hospital setting it is important that those caring for them do not see this as a failure, but rather that they are ensuring that the person receives the best possible care from those who are able to meet their health care needs as the end of their life approaches (Macmillan Cancer Support and Marie Curie Cancer Care, 2013).

Uncertainty over roles and poor communication can contribute to the breakdown of partnership working between health and care organisations (Kirkendall et al, 2012). Social care staff should have regular forums to ask questions regarding how to manage the physical and healthcare needs of the person they are supporting. Equally, healthcare professionals may not be as skilled in understanding how the person is affected by their autism and may require care staff to help them develop an understanding of the person that enables them to best recognise and respond to the person's needs and wishes. It is important to ensure that support roles are clearly defined between healthcare and social care staff so that everyone is aware of the responsibilities of their role.

Pause for thought…

It is vitally important that social care staff and healthcare professionals work closely together to provide the best possible care for the person with a life-limiting illness.

Changes to familiar environments

There may be changes required to support environments to enable the person to remain within their own home. This is likely to include changes in the form of:

- equipment and aids
- adaptations to existing space and layout
- requirement for a variety of healthcare staff to come in and out of the environment.

Early consideration of how the environment may have to be adapted enables best possible preparation. For example there may be a requirement for use of hoists, wheelchairs or monitors as the person's terminal illness progresses. Health teams and **occupational therapists** can assist in ensuring the correct aids and equipment are available to provide the appropriate level of care within the person's home.

Managers of care services should ensure that care staff are appropriately trained to use any aids and equipment that falls into their support remit.

> "NHS Boards should ensure that rapid access is available to appropriate equipment required for the care of those wishing to die at home from any advanced progressive condition."
>
> (Scottish Government, 2008, Action 10)

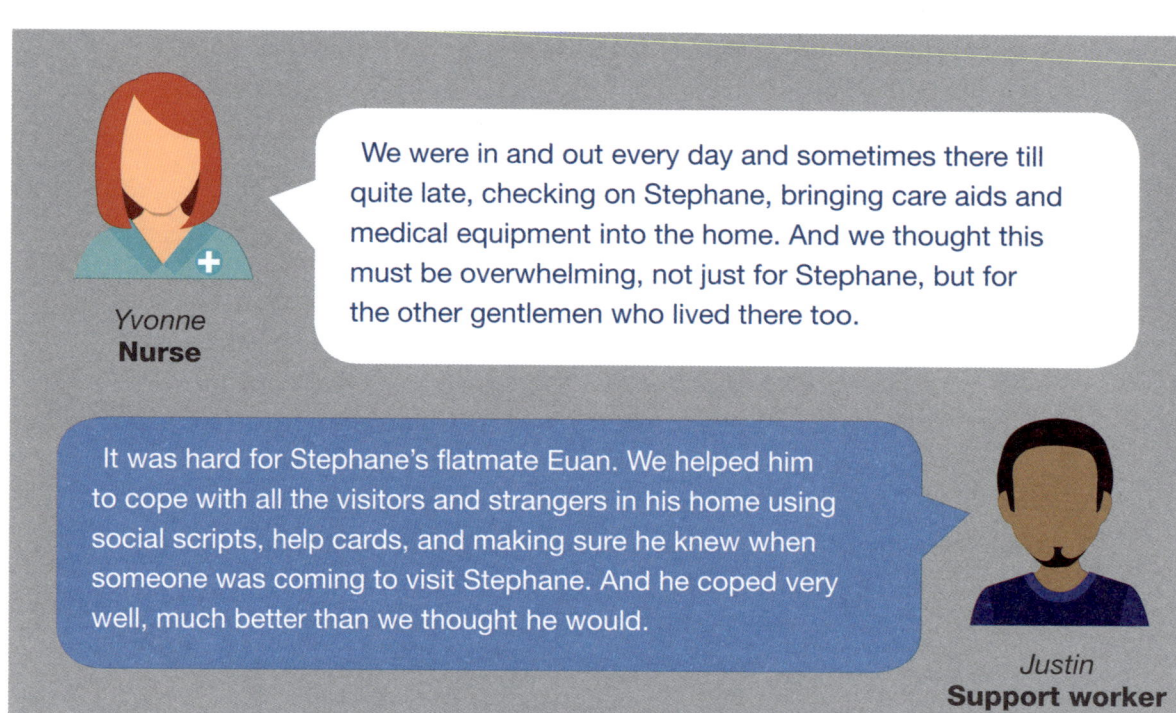

Yvonne
Nurse

We were in and out every day and sometimes there till quite late, checking on Stephane, bringing care aids and medical equipment into the home. And we thought this must be overwhelming, not just for Stephane, but for the other gentlemen who lived there too.

It was hard for Stephane's flatmate Euan. We helped him to cope with all the visitors and strangers in his home using social scripts, help cards, and making sure he knew when someone was coming to visit Stephane. And he coped very well, much better than we thought he would.

Justin
Support worker

Changes to familiar environments and the fact that unfamiliar people may need to come in and out of their homes may be challenging for a person on the autism spectrum. It may also present difficulties in shared support environments due to the changes required to carry out the physical and healthcare needs of the person with a life-limiting illness in their home.

Understanding how an individual learns and takes in new information enables teams to communicate and work through issues of changes effectively. Use of written and pictorial supports might help to provide explanations of what is happening, where, by whom and why.

At the end of life

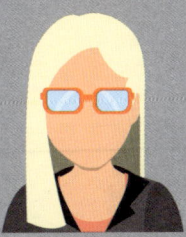

Valerie
Manager

There was a change in Stephane as the end approached. He became increasingly thin and withdrawn and we became very aware of the changes in his breathing. As his illness progressed some of the earlier challenges of his autism started to take a back seat and he became accepting of all the care and support we were giving him. That was very different to what we had seen earlier in his illness.

We spoke to the team before Stephane died about the various ways it might happen. We spoke through the possible eventualities and what to expect at the end of his life. It was important to prepare them for what to expect.

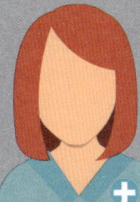

Yvonne
Nurse

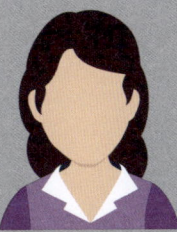

Kirsty
Keyworker

Would I be able to deal with a dead body, that was something I worried about. But I did, because it was still Stephane. Even after he died and the doctor had been in to verify the death, we still had to care for him. I wanted to make him look presentable. These were things I could do when he was alive, and I thought why should it be different now he's dead. If you really care about a person you find the strength from somewhere to do those things that worry you.

During the practitioner workshops one of the most cited fears amongst support staff was whether or not they could cope being the staff member on duty when the person with autism they were supporting died.

Chapter 1: **Physical**

> **Pause for thought...**
>
> Professional support and advice should be sought from healthcare staff about what can be typically expected at the end of a person's life to help prepare individuals and their care staff for the various eventualities.

Some of the things that care staff might typically expect to observe as a person approaches the end of their life include: changes to breathing, confusion and restlessness, decline of senses, loss of bladder or bowel control, skin on hands and feet feeling increasingly cool to touch, loss of consciousness or awareness of those around them.

When the person dies the person supporting them may expect the following to happen:

> *"Sometimes the person will give several outward pants as their heart and lungs stop. Others may give a long out-breath followed quite a few seconds later by what seems another intake of breath. This may be repeated for several minutes, which can be alarming if you are not ready for it. However, this is only the lungs expelling air.*
>
> *There will be no pulse.*
>
> *Skin tone alters and the facial expression changes, or loosens. You may not feel you recognise the person anymore. Some people look remarkably at peace.*
>
> *There is a notion of no-one being 'home'."*

(Dying Matters, 2015)

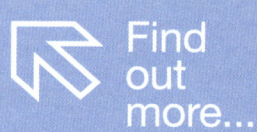

Find out more...

Changes in breathing towards end of life

Marie Curie's website has a short video designed to inform those caring for people at the end of their life about what to expect in changes to the person's breathing.

www.mariecurie.org.uk

An **event of death protocol** and care plan should be drawn up and shared with support staff prior to the end of a person's life. This should detail what is expected of care staff in the event of the person with autism's death. Protocols should be discussed and agreed with local health services.

A protocol might typically include:

- Instructions regarding the body
- Who to contact to verify the death
- Information relating to the individual's personal wishes as per their support plan – this should include any cultural or religious beliefs
- Who needs to be notified and by whom
- Support contingencies for the staff team and other service users in shared accommodation
- Contact information for funeral services
- Reporting instructions (such as completion of incident report to accurately record events, notifications to social work and the Care Inspectorate)

Peaceful, Pain Free and Dignified

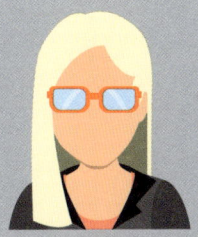

Valerie
Manager

Stephane's last days with us were really very emotional, seeing him so weak and lose all his strength like that. Fortunately his mum was able to be with him at his bedside when he passed away. She wanted to say a prayer in French and we all held hands.

I was glad to be at his side and I held his hand right to his death. My finger was on his pulse and I could feel his pulse stop. His face looked so at peace.

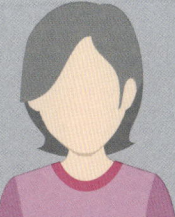

Marian
Mum

It is important to consider in advance who will need to be notified in the event of the death and who is the best person to do that. For example, the GP, NHS 24 or out-of-hours service will need to be notified so that a doctor can verify the death and issue the death certificate. The funeral director, relevant care staff and care managers will need to be contacted, and of course families and the important people in the person's life. If family members are not present at the time of the person's death it is important to agree in advance on a protocol for notifying them that meets their expectations and wishes. Local health and police authorities will have their own local procedures to be followed.

If the individual lives in shared accommodation then a protocol/support plan for informing housemates should also be agreed in advance and followed in the event of death.

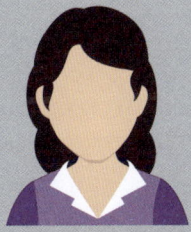

Kirsty
Keyworker

We gave Euan a help card that explained in a very practical way what he could expect to happen on the day Stephane died. It was just a few lines with bullet points on a card that fitted in his wallet, but this was what Euan needed. He needed that reassurance and explanation to be with him throughout Stephane's illness.

Chapter 1: **Physical** 47

Physical: final thoughts

The emphasis on delivery of appropriate physical care and support following diagnosis of life-limiting illness seems to have traditionally focused on the role of healthcare professionals. Their role is essential in managing pain and symptom control to ensure the person is as comfortable as possible as they near the end of their life, but for people on the autism spectrum who face barriers to appropriate care and treatment it is imperative that they are supported by people who understand them as an individual and recognise how the complexities of their autism affect how they will respond to care and consultation.

> *"A shared desire to cooperate does not appear to be sufficient to guarantee effective collaboration. Focused efforts should be directed at building relationships between intellectual disability and palliative care organisations in order to ensure equity of access and delivery of high quality palliative care services."*

(Ryan et al, 2010)

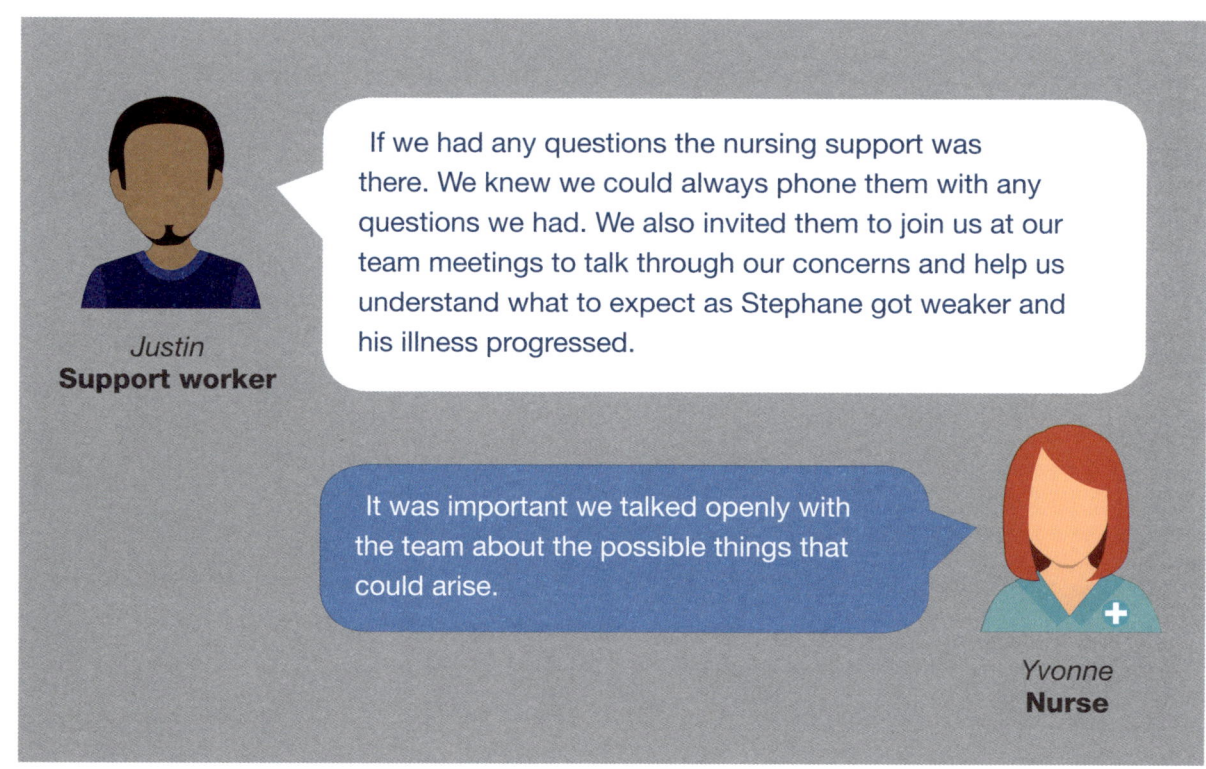

D'Astous and colleagues propose that it is not necessarily the impact of a person's autism that presents barriers to engagement, but rather the often exclusionary nature of societal attitudes, systems and structures (D'Astous, 2014). It is only with shared objectives and cooperation between health and social care teams that we can deliver truly person centred palliative care. Further linking between social care organisations and palliative care teams enables us to pool resources, knowledge and experience that breaks down barriers.

Social communication difficulties and differences in the way people on the autism spectrum experience and relate to the world around them make it more likely that others might make decisions regarding care and support for them, without the appropriate consultation, perceiving them to lack capacity to be involved in those decisions. In the *Handbook of Palliative Care* (2012) Faull and colleagues write of the balance between individual and professional autonomy in the field of palliative care, recognising that where previously decision making in palliative care lay in the hands of the healthcare clinicians there is now a move towards palliative and end of life care that is 'assisted rather than instructed' by the professional. It is through the support and inclusion of the individual themselves, and those who understand how they make choices and communicate their aspirations for their care, we can balance the professional knowledge and clinical experience of healthcare practitioners with the individual autonomy of people on the autism spectrum at the end of their life.

Physical

Discussion points for care teams

- What are some of the challenges in identifying and communicating symptoms of illness in the individuals on the autism spectrum you know and support? What implications might this have for diagnosis and treatment?

- Consider the ability to consent to medical treatment and interventions for the individuals with autism you know and support. Are there any issues of capacity or barriers to self advocacy that require support and consideration?

- What kind of issues might have to be considered regarding care at home or in a hospice? What supports would be required to enable the individual with autism you know or support to stay in their home? What support would be required in the event of a hospital or hospice admission?

At the end of each chapter there is a completed support map and a separate blank template. You can download the blank templates from www.bild.org.uk/supportmapping

Physical: support mapping for care teams

Palliative and end of life care inevitably involves supporting the person diagnosed with a life-limiting condition to cope with the physical implications of their illness. The person may require support to cope with distressing symptoms, get relief from pain, and manage physical changes in themselves as a result of their illness. It involves working very closely with healthcare professionals to ensure the individual is as comfortable and pain free as possible in end of life.

How can we support the person to remain in their home?

What are the challenges in identifying and communicating symptoms of illness for the person you support?

The DisDAT (Disability Distress Assessment Tool) could be helpful

Support required

Environmental and moving and handling assessments to be completed by care team with support from health and safety officer. Multi-agency working and preparation between health and social care.

Any adaptations required

Changes to layout within flat currently sufficient to manage changing support needs. Advice and reassessment from OT as required.

Aids and equipment required

Bed, wheelchair, medication storage updates, zimmer frame, catheter, syringe driver, bath chair, 'just in case' meds

Advice can be sought from Hospice UK, an occupational therapist, your GP and community palliative care team.

Marie Curie and Macmillan's 'End of Life: a guide' could be helpful

Do the care team feel informed and prepared regarding the physical symptoms and support required?

What can we do to help? (key strategies)

Use of pain assessment tools such as DisDAT (disability distress assessment tool) and Abbey pain scales

Meeting with nursing team to discuss implications for pain management and symptom control

Area of support: Inability to distinguish between and articulate different types of pain

What can we do to help? (key strategies)

Consultation with GP and nursing teams around treatment solutions eg use of cream to numb skin in preparation for taking bloods

Area of support: Dislike of needles and particular forms of medication

What can we do to help? (key strategies)

Completion of sensory assessment to inform strategies and supports. Advice from nurses about options to overcome discomfort and minimise anxieties/direct contact

Area of support: Dislike of touch and particular textures on skin

What can we do to help? (key strategies)

Use of photographs and pictorial information to prepare Stephane for changes to home environment and new aids/equipment

What can we do to help? (key strategies)

Use of social scripts and visual planners to inform expectations of appointments/consultations

Use of hospital passport and links with learning disability liaison nurse to inform reasonable adjustments in clinical settings

Area of support: Requirement for aids and equipment at home

Area of support: Unclear expectations about what to expect from consultations

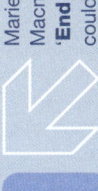
Stephane

Care planning

What are the particular support issues and challenges to managing the physical and healthcare needs of the person you are supporting? What strategies and supports can be put in place to overcome any barriers?

Where an individual is considered to lack capacity to make certain decisions regarding their care and treatment...

Consider the capacity of the person you support to consent to medical treatment and interventions? Have you discussed any identified issues with individuals, families, staff, friends and health teams?

The Mental Welfare Commission's 'Right to Treat' could be helpful

Who should be involved in decisions regarding the person's care and treatment?

Stephane's rights and individual autonomy should be respected at all times.

Stephane has a Section 47 Adults with Incapacity Certificate in place.

Lead health clinicians

Stephane's mother must always be involved in decisions regarding his care

What support measures can we put in place to enable the person to take a more active role in decision making?

Stephane's comprehension and communication difficulties have a significant impact on his ability to self advocate and make decisions regarding his care and treatment.

Attempts should always be made to provide explanations that are appropriate to his understanding, level of coping and capacity to make decisions regarding his care and support

Verbal information should be backed up with visual communication and use of social scripts and stories.

Who are the key health professionals involved?

Name	Role
Yvonne Community palliative care nurse specialist	Nursing care, advice on pain and symptom control, practical and emotional support for patient and care team
Dr Brodie GP	Regular review of patient symptoms and care needs, referrals for specialist support and assistance from primary healthcare teams, review and prescription of medication
Dr McAdam Consultant	Consultant oncologist – diagnosis, scans, palliative care support, ethical consideration of treatment and care pathways
Anna District nurse	Support to manage symptoms and care needs at home

Consider protocols and communication systems that will strengthen joint working with health teams.

Physical: support mapping for care teams

Palliative and end of life care inevitably involves supporting the person diagnosed with a life-limiting condition to cope with the physical implications of their illness. The person may require support to cope with distressing symptoms, get relief from pain, and manage physical changes in themselves as a result of their illness. It involves working very closely with healthcare professionals to ensure the individual is as comfortable and pain free as possible in end of life.

How can we support the person to remain in their home?

Support required

Aids and equipment required

Any adaptations required

Advice can be sought from Hospice UK, an occupational therapist, your GP and community palliative care team.

> Marie Curie and Macmillan's **'End of Life: a guide'** could be helpful

Do the care team feel informed and prepared regarding the physical symptoms and support required?

> What are the challenges in identifying and communicating symptoms of illness for the person you support?
>
> The DisDAT (Disability Distress Assessment Tool) could be helpful

Area of support — What can we do to help? (key strategies)

Area of support — What can we do to help? (key strategies)

Area of support — What can we do to help? (key strategies)

Area of support — What can we do to help? (key strategies)

Area of support — What can we do to help? (key strategies)

Name

Care planning

What are the particular support issues and challenges to managing the physical and healthcare needs of the person you are supporting? What strategies and supports can be put in place to overcome any barriers?

Who should be involved in decisions regarding the person's care and treatment?

> Consider the capacity of the person you support to consent to medical treatment and interventions? Have you discussed any identified issues with individuals, families, staff, friends and health teams?

Where an individual is considered to lack capacity to make certain decisions regarding their care and treatment...

What support measures can we put in place to enable the person to take a more active role in decision making?

> The Mental Welfare Commission's **'Right to Treat'** could be helpful

Who are the key health professionals involved?

Name	Role

Consider protocols and communication systems that will strengthen joint working with health teams.

Chapter 2:
Psychological

Receiving a diagnosis of life-limiting illness is a psychologically challenging experience for the person diagnosed and for those closely involved in their life and care. They will have to come to terms with the implications of their illness and establish their wishes and aspirations for the end of their life. For a person on the autism spectrum this may be further complicated by differences in how they process and understand information and particularly for those who have difficulty labelling and articulating their thoughts and feelings.

There are many sources of information, support and counselling for the emotional and psychological implications of being diagnosed with a life-limiting illness and for those who know and support them who are facing issues of loss and bereavement. Exploring the thoughts, perspectives and feelings of an individual on the autism spectrum going through such a significant period of change and loss may be significantly more challenging due to a number of considerations.

We asked support staff working in autism services what some of the challenges were for the individuals on the autism spectrum they know and support. The challenges most commonly cited were:

- difficulty identifying and labelling feelings
- difficulty managing emotional regulation
- communication barriers to expressing thoughts and feelings
- poor conceptual understanding of illness and death
- difficulty adjusting to change and managing transitions
- difficulty planning for the future as a barrier to successfully conveying wishes and plans for the end of their life
- susceptibility of people on the autism spectrum to heightened stress and anxiety
- lack of specialist counselling and psychological support services experienced in working with people on the autism spectrum
- the emotional and psychological resilience of autism support staff unaccustomed to exploring issues of palliative and end of life care with those they support

Pause for thought...

How would these factors affect how you supported an individual on the autism spectrum to cope emotionally and psychologically from diagnosis of a life-limiting illness through to the end of their life?

Stephane's story

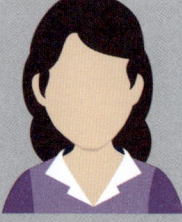

Kirsty
Keyworker

> With his autism and his learning disability I don't think that Stephane fully understood his illness and the concept of death and dying, that he would no longer be here.

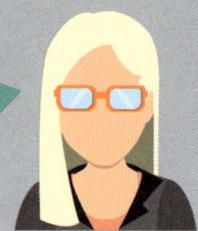

Valerie
Manager

> He understood there was something going on in his body, and we had to very carefully consider how we communicated his illness to him. We didn't want to frighten him or choose words that lacked meaning for him. As a team we looked at social stories to help him understand what would happen, and talking mats to find out what his wishes were, but it was very difficult to fully assess his understanding of what was happening to him.

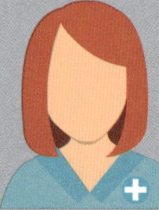

Yvonne
Nurse

> His agitation, his pain, his weight loss, his fatigue. A typical patient can cope with these things, but I thought how do I explain what's happening is normal to someone who doesn't understand so much of the world around them.

In *Palliative Care, Social Work and Service Users*, Beresford and colleagues speak of the field of palliative care as tending to be medically led and burdened by the taboos and difficulties of death thus affecting user involvement and participation. They therefore acknowledge that in the field of palliative and end of life care this creates pressures on participation: *"offering a voice is not the same as accessing people's own voices"* (Beresford et al, 2006).

Accessing the voice of the individuals on the autism spectrum we know and support is the only way we can deliver truly person centred outcomes for individuals across all areas of their life, including in their death. This involves having meaningful conversations that recognise the complexities of how the person's autism affects their communication and how they process information about their diagnosis and the implications of their illness.

Supporting understanding

It is important that the person diagnosed with a life-limiting illness has someone available whom they know and trust to support them to understand their diagnosis. Working with individuals with autism, possibly with a learning disability and communication difficulties, it can be particularly challenging to assess their comprehension and appraisal of the prognosis and to enable open discussion and expression of feeling.

Where there are significant problems assessing a person's understanding and processing of the information being communicated to them it could be useful to involve support from multi-disciplinary teams:

- A **psychologist** might be able to help explore the person's thinking style and reactions to news of life-limiting illness.
- A **speech and language therapist** might be able to work with the individual and their support team to review the way in which news is communicated to support understanding.

Difficult conversations

The language used to discuss serious illness and death is often strewn with metaphor and indirect use of language, culturally considered to be more appropriate to the emotive subject matter. Similarly to bereavement, when supporting an individual with autism to understand the terminology used in palliative and end of life care it is preferable to use simple and factual language (Allison, 1992) or language that has particular meaning and significance to the person. It is also important to establish in what terms death and illness have previously been explained so as not to cause confusion by conveying contradictory information.

Pause for thought...

Does the person with autism you are supporting have a conceptually full understanding of illness and death?

Will they require time to process the information given to them?

What is the best way to communicate important nformation to that person?

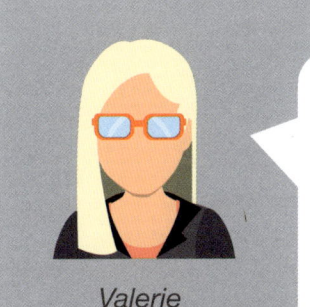

Valerie
Manager

I remember speaking to a family who had explained the anticipated death of a grandparent to their daughter with autism as 'going in the bin'. It seemed so blunt, but to their daughter that was how she understood that something or someone important wasn't coming back. It helped her to understand that death was final. It really demonstrates that need to know the person and how they think.

Breaking bad news challenges what is comfortable to us all for a multitude of societal and personal reasons. The added responsibility of ensuring the language and means of communication used when conveying bad news to a person on the autism spectrum, who may have a different way of processing and understanding information, was cited as a significant concern for staff teams during our practitioner workshops. In addition to a lack of experience communicating news of this nature, care staff may require support as they balance their professional responsibilities with their own emotional responses to the news (Tuffrey-Wijne, 2012).

In shared support environments care staff may also have a responsibility to support the understanding of the person's immediate peer group. Support staff dealing with the emotional responses and care needs of the person with a life-limiting illness may instinctively want to shield other residents from difficult news to minimise distress (Oswin, 1991). However, it is equally important that they have the same support to address their understanding of death and illness and ensure their emotional coping needs are met too.

In *Understanding Death and Illness and What They Teach about Life* (2008), Catherine Faherty addresses the relationship between illness, ageing and death in a resource designed to be accessed both by people on the autism spectrum and practitioners supporting them. Resources like this help address differences in understanding and expectations, exploring many of the questions that arise in response to the subject matter that practitioners may otherwise be reluctant to address, opening up an important dialogue.

Irene Tuffrey-Wijne has endeavoured to develop *"a new model for breaking bad news to people with intellectual disabilities"* that recognises that breaking bad news is not an event it is a process (Tuffrey-Wijne, 2012). This will be equally applicable to working with people on the autism spectrum as support staff work with the individual to build a *"framework of knowledge"* (around death and illness and their own prognosis). This is not something achieved in one event or conversation, but recognises the need to take an exploratory approach to establishing someone's understanding of the complexity of the news and developing their knowledge and understanding in a non-prescriptive or linear way.

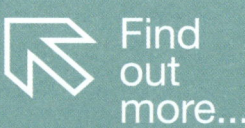

Find out more...

Understanding Death and Illness and What they Teach About Life

A book exploring issues of death and illness for people on the autism spectrum (Faherty, 2008). It is designed to be used both by individuals on the autism spectrum and those supporting them.

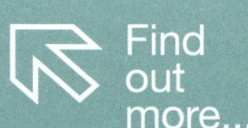

Find out more...

www.breakingbadnews.org

Irene Tuffrey-Wijne

A website offering guidance on how best to break bad news to people with a learning disability.

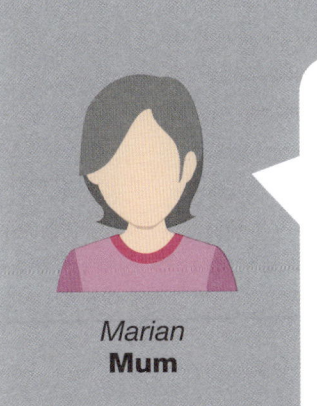

Marian
Mum

> Stephane had experienced grief and loss in his life, firstly when his beloved father passed away. Stephane was at the funeral, and when I explained his father was with Jesus in heaven, Stephane would point to the sky.
>
> He was very fond of cats and loved the feel of their fur. He was devastated at the loss of the cats and I remember him being very quiet and grieving for them. This really affected Stephane for some time.

ARCH (ask, repeat, check and help)

The ARCH model is designed to be a framework for communicating bad news to individuals with a learning disability and might be helpful to think about when framing difficult conversations with individuals on the autism spectrum around diagnosis and prognosis (Read, 2006).

Ask:
- Find out what the person already knows
- Use simple questions to elicit information
- Find out what the person wants to know

Repeat and clarify:
- Be prepared to go over information time and time again, and use a different medium (eg books, photographs)
- Simplify language if necessary
- Actively listen
- Be guided by the individual

Check level of understanding:
- Explore what the person understands (cognitively); what they have 'taken in'
- Explore potential impact
- Go back to previous stage if necessary
- Be guided by the individual

Help individual express feelings:
- Encourage expression; acknowledge feelings and give constructive feedback; help person to describe feelings; explore what they feel they might need next
- Explore future support options
- Follow up where necessary

It is important to consider giving individuals on the autism spectrum adequate processing time, as they may require to think through what has been communicated to them before they are able to respond or engage in any follow up. This may take time and patience and a consistent person they trust to work through the complexity of such important news.

People on the autism spectrum may have a unique outlook or perspective on their own illness and prognosis, or indeed the broader themes of death and illness when explored in conversations with their carers and support staff. It is important that each person's views are valued and respected. Questions in the ARCH framework such as 'find out what the person wants to know' might throw up unexpected questions – it might be a surprising aspect of the change and loss ahead that is of particular concern or worry to that person, or unclear in their thoughts. Where support is required to help a person develop a cognitive appreciation of an aspect of their illness or prognosis, then careful consideration should be given to how that is communicated and by whom.

Care teams should document the communication used and responses given to ensure consistency of message and clarity should the individual initiate a follow-up conversation regarding what has been communicated to them. Updates to communication passports, care plans and other key documents are required to reflect the work done in appraising the person's understanding of their illness and how best to support their cognitive and emotional needs at a time of such significant news.

Challenging 'habits of thought'

> "It's very hard to learn the lesson that things don't and can't last forever. Something that has taken me a very long time to grasp is the idea of mortality. I am always surprised when something comes to an end."
>
> (Lawson, 2000)

The psychiatrist Colin Murray Parkes writes of what he terms *"psychosocial transitions"*. This refers to the transition involved in having to make changes to our assumptions about the world we know following significant change or loss, to challenge our *"habits of thought and behaviour"* (Murray Parkes, 1998).

Approaching death has been described as the *"hidden transition"* (Read, 2006). A diagnosis of life-limiting illness forces the individual diagnosed to acknowledge a whole new set of assumptions about their future and process the implications of their illness whilst facing the inevitability of loss. This psychological transition process can be challenging for any individual, but may be particularly challenging for a person on the autism spectrum whose issues with shifting perspectives and predictive thinking make change and transition particularly difficult. Many people on the autism spectrum are reliant on predictable and habitual interactions and events in day-to-day life to help them make sense of and feel safe in the world around them. If those 'habits of thought' and what is known and familiar are challenged in such a considerable way, this could be particularly stressful or frightening.

Predictive thinking and past experience

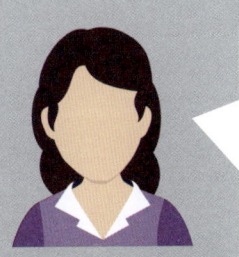

Kirsty **Keyworker**

> Stephane struggled to plan for the future, and was dependent on schedules to help him make sense of his week. If we'd tried to illustrate what was going to happen in three to six months to him that would have been too much for him to cope with. Even more so because he went on to live for a further two and a half years following the diagnosis.
>
> And because he didn't have a full understanding of his prognosis and what that meant, he didn't seem to have the same stress in the earlier stages of his palliative care that you or I would have. Did that affect his prognosis, did that help him live for two and half years instead of the three months he was initially given?

For those people on the autism spectrum who thrive on clear and concrete communication of information, it will not always be possible to offer definitive explanations about the outcome of their diagnosis and the specifics of their prognosis. Whilst death is a universal concept that we all must face in our lives we cannot predict exactly when and how it will occur and this makes it difficult to explain as we would typically do when helping someone prepare for important life events.

Pause for thought...

Whatever the challenges to each individual's thoughts or expectations of their life, it is important to address the subject matter in a way that is appropriate to the individual's style of thinking and reflective of their ability to cope with the information given.

For individuals whose conceptual understanding of aspects of past, present and future may be impaired, it could be distressing to speak of expected death too far in advance (Clements and Zarkowska, 2000). With other people on the autism spectrum the focus of their concerns will tend to be less about the future and more on ruminating over unresolved incidents and episodes of grief from their past (Tantum, 2012). It is important to recognise that previous experiences of change and loss will influence someone's response to news of their prognosis. It has been proposed that this may be particularly true for individuals who have spent their life in residential care and are considered vulnerable to separation, change and loss in their lives (Oswin, 1991).

Experiences of separation, change and loss not only relate to the loss of people but also to homes, objects of significance, health, abilities, social networks and all that is familiar and safe to the person. For people on the autism spectrum whose emotional investment in things that are highly significant to them is not restricted to people (Tantum, 2012) some of those losses will either go unrecognised by those supporting them or they may fail to empathise with the extent of the loss. A developed understanding of how a person has responded to other periods of change and loss in their lives should help care teams put in informed strategies and supports in the event of news of life-limiting illness.

Processing information

Differing information processing styles in people on the autism spectrum may mean they struggle with issues of delayed or fragmented processing. If someone typically experiences delayed processing it is important to give them time to digest important information. We must also remember not to take reactions to difficult news at face value as there may be a delayed reaction to processing thoughts and in turn expression of emotions such as fear or anger.

There is a particular concern for individuals who have difficulty with fragmented processing or attend to atypical stimulus in any given situation or exchange. There is a possibility that they will not process all of the important information being communicated to them, or that they may take in a fragment of the communication that might be out of context or fail to be the most salient piece of information they require to process. It is therefore important to engage in follow-up

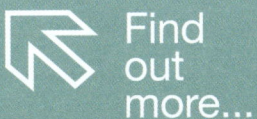

Find out more...

CHANGE Cancer Series

Palliative Care, End of Life Care and Bereavement

An accessible series of books available in 'easy read' and 'for carers' formats that give support and information to people with learning disabilities and their carers through terminal illness, dying and bereavement.

Available via the Macmillan Cancer Support website:

www.macmillan.org.uk

---

conversations that gauge the fullness of the person's understanding of what has been communicated. It might also be useful to split communication into smaller, more easily processed portions of information.

Resources such as Change's 'CHANGE Cancer' series of accessible books for people with learning disabilities and their carers can be valuable sources of reference that enable carers to explore themes of life-limiting illness and palliative care in a very accessible fashion. This can be used to inform difficult discussions and act as a source of information that can be used and revisited to reinforce understanding and expectations.

It is important to recognise that people on the autism spectrum are not just adversely challenged by the differences in typical thinking characteristics of their autism. This can also bring fresh perspectives and informative outlooks on life that broaden the thinking of those who know and support them. It may be that the person on the autism spectrum you know or support has a particular way of rationalising or reasoning the information given to them that helps them manage some of the challenges and stresses of such news in a way that other people might not, or that 'typical' stressors are not of concern to the person because they lack significance in their life.

The answers to these questions can be used to:

- tailor information and communication to be reflective of the person's thinking and learning style
- motivate engagement in important discussions and support understanding by making information relatable
- prioritise the information being communicated based on the person's needs and not what we presume is appropriate based on our own feelings and experiences

Pause for thought...

When a person on the autism spectrum we are supporting receives such life-changing news we should take time to stop and understand.

How does the person think about and experience the world around them?

How do they learn and take in new information?

What is important to them in their life?

Chapter 2: **Psychological**

Emotions and feelings

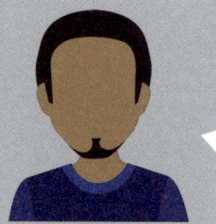

Justin
Support worker

> It was upsetting to see when he was in pain, or when he wanted us or the nurses not to do something. To see him getting thinner and thinner and weaker and weaker, that was difficult to watch.

> The practical side of things is the practical side of things and I think you can do that when it's part of your job. To emotionally detach yourself that's difficult, it was always going to be difficult. But to do your job you had to take a step back and say the best I can do for him is be professional.

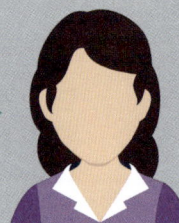

Kirsty
Keyworker

Put your own oxygen mask on first

People on the autism spectrum are frequently represented as having difficulty coping with change and transition. However, we are all creatures of habit, routine and ritual and all of us are subject to the vulnerability and *"disorganisation"* that profound and unforeseen change and loss can bring to our lives (Watts, 2009).

Paid carers cannot be expected to mechanically suppress their emotional response to the news that a person they support has been diagnosed with a life-limiting illness. Professionalism does not equate to dispassion and it is of course natural to find a practice situation such as this emotionally challenging, particularly as a social care worker unaccustomed to providing support of this nature. It is important in any challenging practice situation that care staff take time to address their own coping first to enable them to then support others, to *"put their own oxygen mask on first"* (McCreadie, 2014).

Delivering end of life support can be emotionally demanding on a staff team and they must always have a platform for sharing their feelings, be able to express their fears and have a safe space for voicing a need for help when it is required. It is important that specific consideration is made regarding the emotional support for the care staff (Tuffrey-Wijne, 2012) so that they are equipped to best support the person they are caring for.

> **Pause for thought...**
>
> You will find more information on support for care staff in Chapter 3.

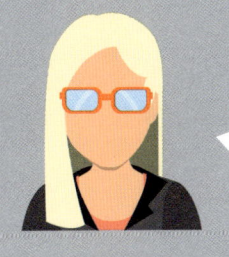

> It was important for us as a support team to come to terms with our own fears and feelings before we could properly support Stephane. We were very fortunate that we could talk openly with each other about how we felt and were there to support each other.

Valerie
Manager

Expressing emotions and labelling feelings

Establishing social support mechanisms and interpreting emotional states can be more difficult for people on the autism spectrum. For individuals who struggle to identify and label their feelings it could prove difficult to provide the correct emotional support in the event of a diagnosis of life-limiting illness. Exploration of emotional states in individuals at the end of their life will always be guided by the pace the person is comfortable with. It is important not to force someone to work through difficulties that they are not ready to resolve, understanding that people will often accept change more readily *"if the walls of their defences against it are taken down brick by brick"* (Wright, 2007).

Wendy Lawson, a writer who is on the autism spectrum, explains that *"emotions are not concrete structures that can be seen, held or organized"* (Lawson, 2000) and this lack of tangibility makes processing and labelling feelings a particular challenge.

Rachel Forrester-Jones and Sarah Broadhurst (2003) suggest that as with any other individual the person with autism may undergo the four stages of bereavement when going through a period of change and loss: denial, anger, despair and adjustment. They then go on to give examples of emotions and presenting behaviours that the individual with autism may exhibit throughout these four stages, such as confusion, compulsive or ritualistic behaviour, anxiety, self-harm and difficulty communicating feelings. For some individuals these are not untypical occurrences in day-to-day life, and therefore it is possible that symptoms of grief may be overlooked or attributed to everyday stressors and issues. Equally we will often also see individuals on the autism spectrum use withdrawal as an attempt at resolving distress, and therefore there exists a risk of this coping mechanism being misinterpreted as indifference or lack of emotion (Clements and Zarkowska, 2000).

Pause for thought...

Not outwardly showing or typically expressing emotions such as fear and grief, does not mean that a person does not experience them.

Emotional regulation is the process of balancing our emotional responses appropriately to the demands of the situation, in accordance with social norms and in a way that protects our wellbeing. It also allows us to *"regain our balance once the difficult moment has passed... To stay in just the right zone"* (Garland, 2014). If a person on the autism spectrum has difficulty with emotional regulation then their responses are more likely to appear out of context or disproportionate to the event. Individuals who struggle with regulation or emotional sensitivity may also experience emotions out of context (Isanon, 2008), or in such an overwhelming manner they struggle to cope.

The use of art therapy and creative expression with individuals on the autism spectrum could serve as a platform for expression of emotion and exploration of personal feelings. This may be preferable to other means of intervention because of its indirect and therefore less socially challenging nature.

Dying, Bereavement and the Healing Arts (Bolton, 2007) gives examples of how using an expressive approach to visual and written imagery can help professionals, patients and carers to explore and represent a person's life.

Anxiety, agitation and distress

In her chapter 'Emerging pathways for the study of stress, coping and autism' in *Stress and Coping in Autism*, Kathleen Morgan writes of the behavioural and biological similarities between people who experience heightened levels of stress and many individuals on the autism spectrum, both presenting as:

> *"socially withdrawn, easy to arouse and difficult to soothe. They are often hyper vigilant, unable to sleep well, or unable to pay attention. They may make poor decisions and show impairment in their working memory. They frequently engage in repetitive and sometimes self-injurious behaviour."*

(Morgan in Baron et al, 2006)

It is understandable that the challenges of making sense and meaning of a world you don't feel you fit into can be a source of significant stress for a person on the autism spectrum (McCreadie and McDermott, 2014) and it has been proposed that up to 60 per cent of people on the autism spectrum are perceived to have anxiety related issues or disorders (Baranger and Sullings, 2013). For individuals already at high risk of experiencing heightened stress and anxiety in day-to-day life it is important to consider how as support teams we can work to minimise the stresses and fears of living with a life-limiting illness. A programme of holistic support and interventions that recognises not just symptom control but the relationship between physical and psychological wellbeing is essential in promoting peace at the end of a person's life. Mind-body techniques that encourage relaxation and mindfulness can help address some of the psychological and emotional issues associated with palliative and end of life care (Faull et al, 2012).

There may be many ways that the individual diagnosed with a life-limiting illness expresses distress or agitation as a result of their illness. It may not just be through obvious signs of distress, but also through changes in typical presentation, withdrawal, changes in appetite and sleeping patterns, or through behaviours that others find challenging. It may be hard to identify these and in some cases separate them from the physical symptoms and side effects of illness and pain for individuals who struggle to articulate their feelings. This is why we need to take time to understand the nuances of an individual's *"language of distress"* (Rehal, 2013).

> *"An increase in activity due to distress may be interpreted as challenging behaviour, while reduced activity may be wrongly interpreted as someone being quiet and content."*
>
> (Read, 2006)

Emotion thermometer tools © are used in clinical settings to monitor emotional wellbeing and distress in patients. Use of a visual scale to explore stress and emotion may be an appropriate strategy for working with people on the autism spectrum.

Emotion Works © may be useful for teams supporting people on the autism spectrum who struggle to articulate how they are feeling or express this in a non-typical way. The tool employs a component model of emotion to break down how someone is feeling through exploration of sensations, language, influences, behaviours and strategies for regulation.

(You can find out more about these tools at www.emotionthermometers.com and www.emotionworks.org.uk.)

For people on the autism spectrum who report differing experiences of the world around them (Bogdashina, 2011) it follows that their presentation and interactions are likely to be idiosyncratic and difficult to interpret for those who don't know them well. Life-limiting illness will bring additional stresses that may impact on their presentation and wellbeing and could exacerbate pre-existing issues with information processing and emotional regulation. It also follows that whilst there will be common stressors likely to be experienced by people with autism and those who are not on the autism spectrum, individuals with autism may also be distressed by aspects of their illness and prognosis that are not recognised as stressful because the people supporting them find it difficult to relate to the stressor themselves (Twachtman-Cullen in Baron et al, 2006).

The psychological pressures and worries of knowing and supporting someone diagnosed with a life-limiting illness from diagnosis through to their death will also affect others on the autism spectrum who share the person's life and for the care staff supporting the person at the end of their life.

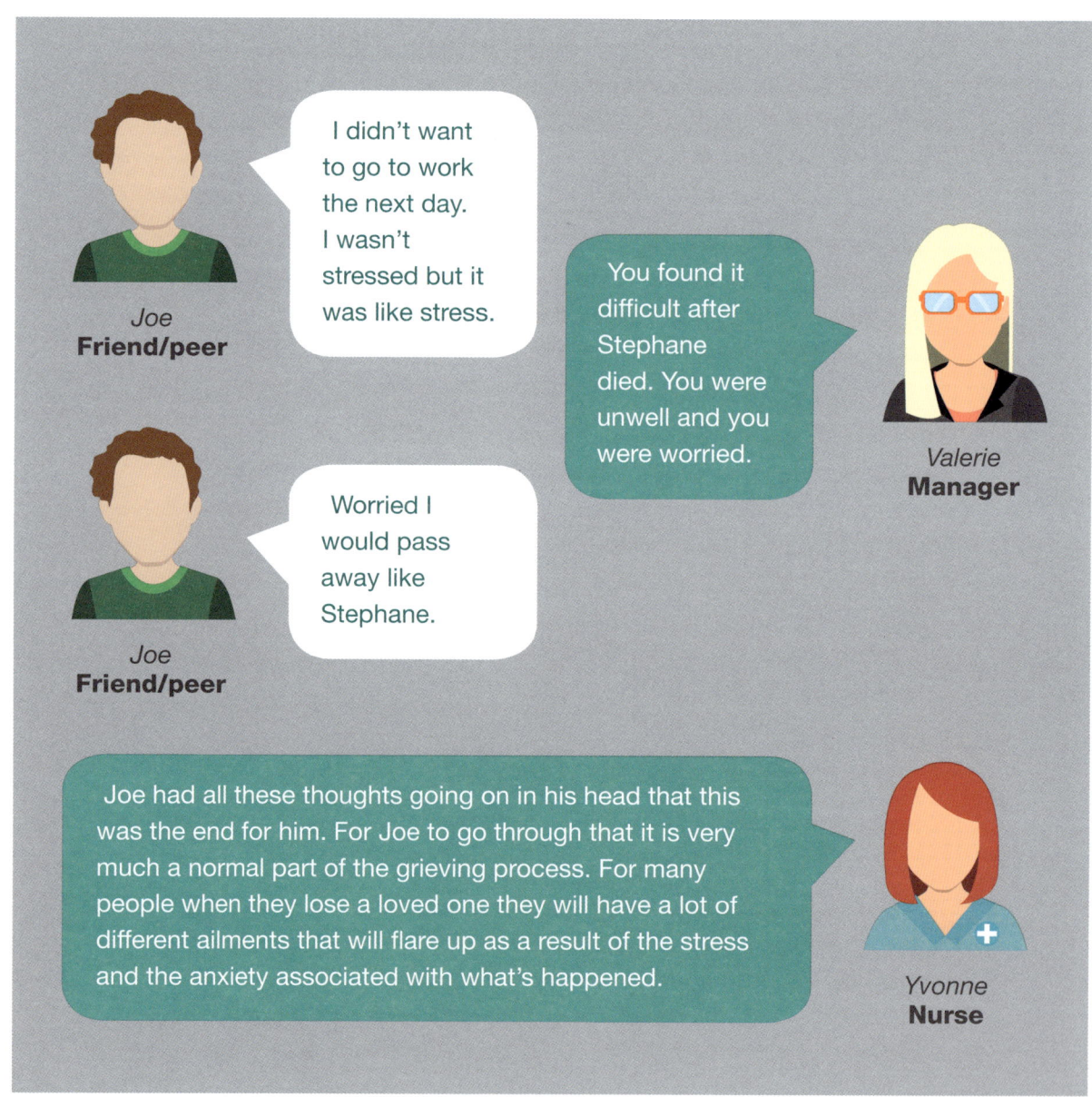

Stress is both transactional and contextual. Whilst the difficulties associated with living on the autism spectrum understandably generate stressors in a person's life; levels of distress and grief are influenced by many different factors such as the perceptions and reactions of others, past experiences, the environment, cultures and beliefs.

It is wrong to indicate that any person or group has a global incapacity to cope with stress (Murray Parkes, 1998). Many people on the autism spectrum can show incredible resilience and strength in the face of adversity and challenge. Perceptions about what is distressing news or a challenging experience will be subjective and very personal to the individual. Once more this demonstrates the importance of support from figures of trust who are knowledgeable about how the person on the autism spectrum they know or support expresses loss of psychological and emotional wellbeing. Also important is support from people who have a developed understanding of what makes the person happy in life and can build in supports based on positive experiences and motivations.

Patient and carer diaries can be used for documenting experiences and feelings for the person diagnosed with a life-limiting illness and those supporting them. Encouraging someone to reflect on what is 'bad about today' promotes an open dialogue about the challenges they are facing, whilst reflecting on what was 'good about today' can help to counter negative feelings and enable teams to plan a person's care built on positive experiences that help promote wellbeing.

Peter Vermeulen advocates an approach to working with people on the autism spectrum that focuses less on negative feelings and events, but instead invests in supports that foster positive feelings and self esteem (Vermeulen, 2014). It is easy in the face of such life-changing news to focus all our attention and supports on the challenges ahead; but at the end of life, as we have needed throughout our lives, there is still a necessity to find happiness and peace within ourselves.

Loss of self ability

It is inevitable that as the person's illness progresses they will become increasingly dependent on the support of health and social care staff to meet their daily needs and carry out aspects of personal care and support that they previously were able to do independently. In addition to a loss of ability to attend to personal care and everyday life skills, there will also be a loss of the ability to engage in important activities, events and routines. This loss of self ability is likely to have psychological implications for the person's wellbeing and require explanation to counter feelings of anger or frustration.

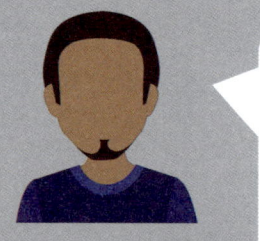

Justin
Support worker

It was difficult as Stephane became more dependent on our physical support as he didn't like people to touch him. But a lot of his frustration came from the fact he had lost the ability to do things he used to do for himself. You could see on his face he still wanted to do it but he just didn't have the energy any more.

There will be people on the autism spectrum who have been dependent on others to take decisions for them regarding their care and treatment throughout their illness. They will also have potentially lacked control over significant decisions affecting them throughout their lives due to a perceived lack of capacity or social communication difficulties, and as with anyone with a life-limiting illness they will have no control over the inevitability of their death. A loss of control over the decisions and outcomes that affect your life can have a significant impact on a person's self esteem and emotional wellbeing. It is important as social care staff that we promote independence and autonomy wherever possible throughout any person's life. We need to be particularly mindful when supporting someone towards the end of their life of the psychological impact of loss of independence and self ability.

Psychological: final thoughts

The psychological consequences of being diagnosed with a life-limiting illness can only be explored through consideration of understanding, insight and emotion.

Inevitably the neurodevelopmental nature of autism spectrum conditions means that the people on the spectrum we know and support may have differing ways of thinking and responding to the world around them. Their emotional literacy and responses may not always be typical, but they will always be human. We have to appreciate that news of this nature and the psychological implications of the ensuing care will often be understood and expressed in a diversity of ways, but all of them grounded in human experience.

The idea of acceptance and an associated sense of peace are often sought by those facing the frightening inevitability of death.

Cynthia Kim is a writer on the autism spectrum who writes of the link between acceptance and wellbeing. She describes the difference that having an explanation about her autism made in terms of self-acceptance, the difference between thinking she was wrong and accepting she was different (Kim, 2014). Similarly for someone on the autism spectrum being asked to accept news of a life-limiting illness, we need to ensure that we engage in a dialogue with the person that supports understanding and provides opportunities for exploring feelings to help in that quest for inner peace and acceptance.

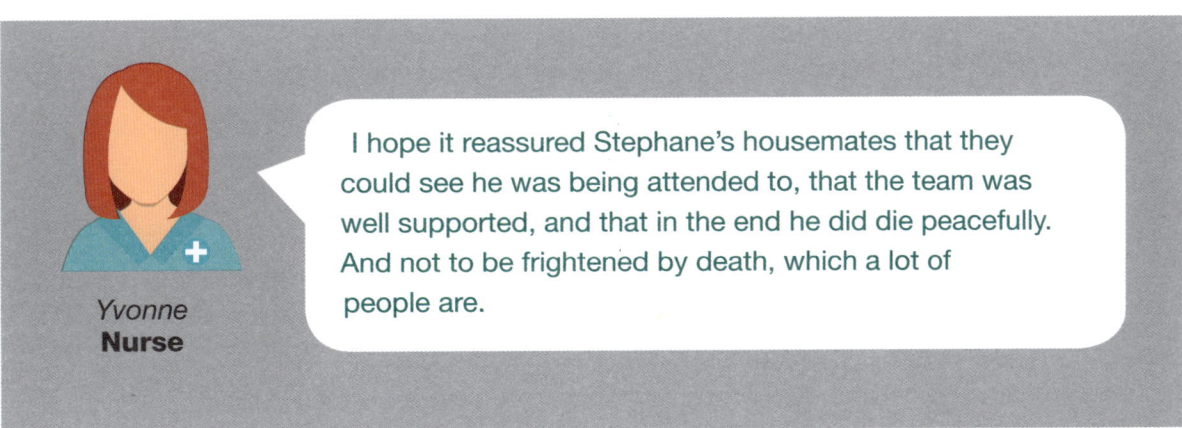

Yvonne
Nurse

I hope it reassured Stephane's housemates that they could see he was being attended to, that the team was well supported, and that in the end he did die peacefully. And not to be frightened by death, which a lot of people are.

Psychological

Discussion points for care teams

- How do the people on the autism spectrum you know/support express feelings of fear, depression, anger? Are they able to label and articulate those feelings?

- How would you best inform a person on the autism spectrum you know or support about their illness/prognosis? Consider explanations and strategies to support understanding and promote emotional wellbeing.

- What might the psychological impact be on the people you know or support following a significant loss of self ability? How would you counter negative feelings arising from an increased dependency on others?

Psychological: support mapping for care teams

Receiving a diagnosis of life-limiting illness is a psychologically challenging experience for the person diagnosed and for those closely involved in their life and care. For a person on the autism spectrum this may be further complicated by differences in how they think and process information, and particularly for those who have difficulty labelling and articulating their thoughts and feelings. The person diagnosed with a life-limiting illness will have to cope with loss of emotional wellbeing as they try to come to terms with the implications of their illness and establish their wishes and aspirations for the end of their life.

Emotions and feelings

What might be the psychological impact on the person following a significant loss of independence and self ability?

Could using **Good About Today/Bad About Today diaries** help someone reflect on how they are feeling and why?

> How does the person you know/support express feelings of fear, depression, anger, acceptance?
> Are they able to label these feelings?
> Do they express them in a typical way?

What was the experience of loss, change or ill health	How did they cope?	What strategies and supports can we put in place to help with future change and loss?
Stephane's father died when he was ten years old	Stephane was close to his father and this was his first real experience of close loss. He appeared to understand with support that his father was 'gone' and accepted relocating him in 'heaven'.	Stephane attended his father's funeral. It was explained to Stephane that his father had 'gone to heaven to be with Jesus'. Consider use of language that Stephane is familiar with. Stephane pointed to the sky to indicate that his father was in heaven – use of gesture to inform communication strategies.
Loss of pet cats	Withdrawn and quiet for period of time, genuine sadness and grief	Buried the family cats as per funeral custom and Stephane required verbal support/closure to understand that he wouldn't see them again, 'gone'.

How does the person you support express their emotions, are they able to label feelings?

Able to verbalise whether something is 'good' or 'bad' but largely unable to label and articulate his feelings.

Expression of emotion through body language and actions.

Stephane requires to be supported by people who have the knowledge and observational skills to read his feelings and the subtleties of his expressions and presentation. (See individual support plan)

How does the person learn and take in new information?

Use of visual supports and schedules helps firm up Stephane's understanding of new information and changes.

Stephane takes cues from his environment, attention to salient information reinforced with pictorial direction or cues such as sounds or tangible objects.

Learns through practical experiences.

Requires encouragement to approach new and unfamiliar things with the help of known motivators.

How has the person coped with previous experiences of change/loss/ill health?

How can we support the staff team to feel confident having 'difficult conversations'

www.breakingbadnews.org could be helpful

Strategies to support understanding/alternative means of communication

Stephane may verbalise that he is 'sore'

Stephane will point to the area that is sore, and can be encouraged to gesture and use his 'help' card

Body language and facial expression can indicate pain. Changes in mood, repetitive movements and changes to skin tone and temperature can all be indicators of pain. Stephane requires support from people who know and understand him to read his expressions and changes in presentation.

Terms and phrases used	Understanding of term
Cancer	Limited understanding of term 'cancer', Stephane understands that he is unwell
Pain	Stephane understands the term 'sore' but is unable to be more descriptive about different forms and levels of pain

Supporting understanding

Will the person have difficulty understanding any aspect of what is being communicated to them?

CHANGE Cancer Series: palliative care, end of life care and bereavement could be helpful

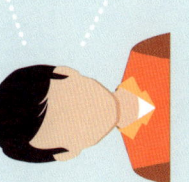

Stephane

Psychological

How can we better understand the thinking style of the person we are supporting?

How will the news of their diagnosis be received and understood?

What is important in the person's life? How can this be used to prioritise information and motivate engagement?

Family – explanations of illness and diagnosis based on prior experiences of change and loss from childhood

Appointments and consultations to be built around time spent on more motivating activities – visiting places of interest, favourite meals, buying favourite magazines.

How can we promote peace and wellbeing to counter stress and agitation?

Places of relaxation: consider comfort within the home, outside of the home, visiting places such as air fields, beaches and churches

Minimise demands within the day – reduce stressors

Activities: 'flow' activities such as drawing, comforting foods, magazines and photographs, consult 'Bliss' therapist about relaxing sensory experiences.

Recognise the importance of consistency and routine within Stephane's day.

Psychological: support mapping for care teams

Receiving a diagnosis of life-limiting illness is a psychologically challenging experience for the person diagnosed and for those closely involved in their life and care. For a person on the autism spectrum this may be further complicated by differences in how they think and process information, and particularly for those who have difficulty labelling and articulating their thoughts and feelings. The person diagnosed with a life-limiting illness will have to cope with loss of emotional wellbeing as they try to come to terms with the implications of their illness and establish their wishes and aspirations for the end of their life.

Emotions and feelings

> What might be the psychological impact on the person following a significant loss of independence and self ability?

> How does the person you know/support express feelings of fear, depression, anger, acceptance?
> Are they able to label these feelings?
> Do they express them in a typical way?

> How does the person you support express their emotions, are they able to label feelings?

> Could using **Good About Today/ Bad About Today** diaries help someone reflect on how they are feeling and why?

What was the experience of loss, change or ill health	How did they cope?	What strategies and supports can we put in place to help with future change and loss?

How can we support the staff team to feel confident having 'difficult conversations'

www.breakingbadnews.org could be helpful

Terms and phrases used	Understanding of term	Strategies to support understanding/ alternative means of communication

Supporting understanding

> Will the person have difficulty understanding any aspect of what is being communicated to them?

CHANGE Cancer Series: palliative care, end of life care and bereavement could be helpful

- What is important in the person's life? How can this be used to prioritise information and motivate engagement?

- How does the person learn and take in new information?

- How can we promote peace and wellbeing to counter stress and agitation?

Name

Psychological

- How can we better understand the thinking style of the person we are supporting?
- How will the news of their diagnosis be received and understood?

- How has the person coped with previous experiences of change/loss/ill health?

Chapter 3:
Social

People diagnosed with a life-limiting illness are cited as vulnerable to loss of social relationships and networks as a result of the physical and psychological implications of their illness. For individuals on the autism spectrum whose ability to form and sustain social relationships can be particularly complex it is important to consider how they will maintain and in some cases redefine the relationships and interactions they have with the significant people within their life.

Stephane's story

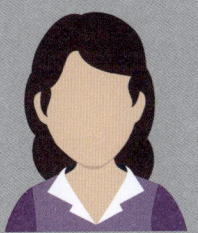

Kirsty
Keyworker

Stephane knew we were trying to help him. I think it was important that he had the same team around him at the end. We had many, many volunteers and offers of support, people wanting to help. But in the last six months of Stephane's life it was the same group of people and he needed that. We understood him, we knew when he was in pain. He was comfortable with us and I think he felt safe with us.

Often social support following diagnosis of a life-limiting illness is defined in very practical terms as assistance with *"getting their affairs in order"* (Department of Health, 2006). For the purposes of this practitioner guide we recognise that staff teams may also be required to provide support to other significant people in the person's life as part of the holistic nature of palliative and end of life care and acknowledge the shared responses and responsibilities amongst all groups of people who have a significant role to play in the person's life and care.

Pause for thought...

What implications does this have for the social support needs of a person on the autism spectrum from diagnosis of a life-limiting illness through to the end of their life?

We asked support staff working in autism services what some of the social challenges were for the individuals on the autism spectrum they know and support. The challenges most commonly cited were:

- social communication challenges affecting interactions with others
- social understanding difficulties affecting a person's ability to form, sustain and understand the rules of relationships
- difficulty intuitively understanding and responding to the emotional responses of others
- relationships can be atypical in nature and therefore not valued accordingly by others
- other people's perceptions about the social motivations of people on the autism spectrum
- meeting the social expectations of the significant people in their lives if their views and aspirations differ
- fear amongst support teams of having to address difficult issues with individuals and the important people in their lives

It is important to understand that social support encompasses a multi-faceted understanding of the relationships and connections between the person on the autism spectrum and all those involved in their life and care. We must acknowledge the need to understand *"the ripple effects of grief on all the components and contexts within which someone lives"* (Beresford et al, 2007).

This requires adaptability of social support and communication on the part of staff teams who find themselves having to be equally comfortable in such roles as: communicating important information to a person on the autism spectrum about their prognosis; talking to distressed family members who want to recount memories and share their aspirations for the future; and liaising with professionals in health and social work regarding practical arrangements for the delivery of support and care packages.

Communication skills amongst support teams are pivotal in the delivery of appropriate and sensitively delivered care (Faull et al, 2012) and staff members' fears and their emotions will inevitably affect their confidence addressing such issues. It is important that each staff member has opportunities to openly reflect about what they will find personally challenging to enable the correct supports and training to be put in place.

Social support for people on the autism spectrum

> *"Perhaps the most hurtful of the myths about autism is the idea that people with the condition are, by nature, asocial and selfish. It's true that social difficulties are a hallmark of the condition and there is plenty of research showing that people with autism struggle with 'theory of mind' (ToM) tasks that involve putting themselves in other people's shoes. However, it's important to realise that ToM involves two elements – a cognitive component and an emotional component. Although people with autism often struggle with the cognitive challenge of taking another person's perspective, there is not necessarily anything lacking in their feelings for other people's joy and pain."*
>
> (Jarrett, 2014)

Individuals on the autism spectrum are often viewed as lacking empathy and emotion due to their social cognition difficulties, but it could equally be argued that there exists a *"double empathy problem"* (Milton, 2014) – people who are not on the autism spectrum often fail to recognise and understand the motivations and intentions of people on the autism spectrum because these differ from what they typically observe and expect from others.

Difficulties with social understanding and communication may mean that the way a person on the autism spectrum interacts with others and endeavours to understand the nuances of social rules and relationships seems atypical when compared to those who are not on the spectrum. Our social motivations and connections with others remain deeply personal and diverse for all of us; but people on the autism spectrum may require additional support to navigate their way through the complexity of social relationships.

One of the ways you may be required to do this is through supporting the person on the autism spectrum to decode the emotional language and responses of those around them at a time of such upsetting news. The role of support teams may not only be to help the person on the autism spectrum to recognise and manage their own responses to their diagnosis and prognosis, but also to recognise and accept the responses of others around them also affected by the news.

There may be a need for the person on the autism spectrum to re-define aspects of their relationships and accept the changing roles of important people in their life following their diagnosis and particularly towards the end of their life. For example, individuals who have been independent in managing their day-to-day care might find it difficult for support staff and family members to provide personal care and physical support to them.

Others who thrive on predictability in their interactions with others may not be prepared for the emotive and qualitatively different responses from people who are close to them in their lives who are struggling with their own thoughts and feelings about the person's illness and prognosis. It may be necessary to prepare the person for the fact that there may be tears, expressions of love, a desire to recall shared memories from the past.

It can be easy to presume that those individuals on the autism spectrum who have particularly profound social communication difficulties are not perceptive to the emotions and responses of those around them. Again, the fact that someone does not respond reciprocally in a typical manner does not mean they are not affected or influenced by the worries, stresses and emotions of those around them.

Such a decline in a person's health understandably compromises their ability and motivation to engage in social events and activities and there exists a risk of loss of social supports and networks that may have played an important role in the person's life prior to their illness. Many people on the autism spectrum struggle to initiate social interaction and activities, or have difficulty with flexible thinking that could impact on their ability to adapt to changing social circumstances. This makes them particularly vulnerable to social losses without support and accommodations. This can be particularly profoundly felt for older people on the autism spectrum, with ageing cited as a trigger for an even higher risk of social exclusion (Baranger and Sullings, 2013).

It is important to find ways to help the person you are supporting to maintain friendships and interests. When the person is no longer physically able to take part in activities that engage their interests or link in with other people, we need to find new ways to share in these and provide positive experiences that help detract from illness and discomfort.

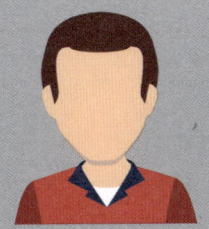

Euan
Housemate

It was a shame for Stephane because he used to enjoy swimming. I can remember years ago he used to be able to go to the transport museum. I showed the staff my pictures of us there. I felt sad for him. I felt sorry for him.

We used photographs, books and magazines to help Stephane maintain his friendships and interests when he became less able to take part in the activities he used to enjoy.

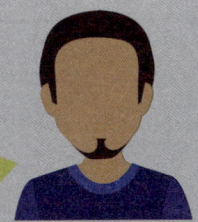

Justin
Support worker

As with emotions, memories and experiences are not concrete things. The person on the autism spectrum you are supporting may need the help of others who know them well and have shared in important moments in their lives to continue that process of sharing and help in the construction of their biography.

It can be useful to consider multi-sensory strategies to help reflect on shared memories and experiences. In addition to the use of visual prompts such as photo-graphs, think about ways to include familiar scents, sounds and textures.

Blackman (2003) advocates the use of the senses as a tool for reminiscence, and this may be particularly important for individuals on the autism spectrum whose sensory perceptual experiences may differ from ours. A particular sensory channel or experience may trigger memories, or perhaps multi-sensory strategies and supports help the person to evoke a fuller picture of what they are being asked to reflect on.

Friends and peers on the autism spectrum

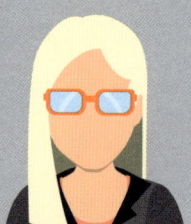

Valerie
Manager

> As the manager of the service I felt quite aware of my responsibilities to the other three people who lived with Stephane. It was important for me to be continually checking how they were coping and I was quite conscious throughout the process that I had to balance the needs of Stephane with the other three gentleman with autism he shared his home and his life with. I wasn't sure if they would cope with the changes in their home, with Stephane's illness, and then of course when he passed away. Thankfully they did and Stephane was able to stay within his home, with the people he knew, the people he had grown and aged with.

In shared support environments there will inevitably be a requirement for care teams to address the support needs of the housemates, residents and peers who know and share in the life of the person with a life-limiting illness. It is important to consider their coping and wellbeing as they go through a period of adjustment and inevitably loss.

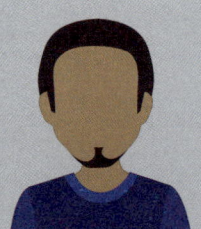

Justin
Support worker

> Stephane's mum would give his flatmate cards to say thank you for his support, and I don't think she realised how much that meant to Euan. It gave him a boost to feel like he was doing well when he was really worried that Stephane was leaving.

> I think it was good Stephane was in his house with people he knew. Euan accepted everything and it must have been very difficult for him, all the coming and going of doctors and nurses in particular. I thought he was admirable.

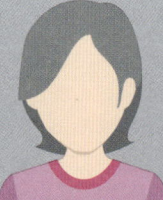

Marian
Mum

Peaceful, Pain Free and Dignified

When considering issues of change and loss, Blackman (2008) encourages practitioners to look for changes in the functioning of the individual. She suggests that the skills and abilities of the person are in danger of being impaired by responses to grief and that their ability to communicate with others is one of these abilities most at risk. Whilst some individuals with autism learn to adapt to loss, others find it particularly difficult. Donna Williams writes of her phobia of forming attachments following early experiences of loss (Williams, 2003), and this social withdrawal is indicative of how negative experiences of grief can have a harmful impact on the individual's wellbeing and personal beliefs.

Carers may overlook signs of stress related to loss (Blackman, 2003) and Maureen Oswin (1991) goes as far as to suggest there may even be a *"denial of feeling"* for people who have learning or communication difficulties. It is therefore imperative care teams are skilled in identifying grief responses in the people they support and have the confidence to enable open discussion to ensure the person has an opportunity to experience grief that in turn enables them to emerge from their loss (Wright, 2007).

The relationships of trust that can be built between service users and practitioners are what enables individuals on the autism spectrum accessing support services to have an outlet for seeking support during periods of loss (Beresford et al, 2007).

The *When someone you know has died...* workbook (Read, 2012) is the outcome of a collaboration between advocacy groups and individuals with learning disabilities in Stoke and Wrexham. It was designed to recognise the value of peer support and learning in the event of loss and bereavement and could be used to open up discussion with people on the autism spectrum going through a period of grief and loss, either on an individual basis or if appropriate in a group setting to enable peer advocacy and support.

It is important that those who have shared in the person's life and are going through a period of loss and adjustment have opportunities to talk through how they are feeling and remember the person who is dying or has died in a way that is appropriate to their needs and wishes.

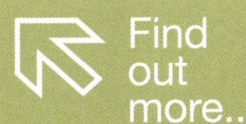

Find out more...

When someone you know has died...

People with learning disabilities supporting each other

This workbook is inspired by the work of a bereavement support group for people with learning disabilities. Through their discussions they developed this peer support booklet to be used by other groups of individuals going through similar experiences.

Access to Learning Disability Healthcare

aldhc.co.uk

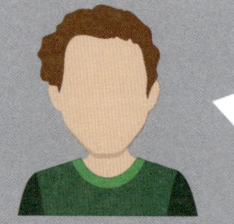

> He liked to talk about aeroplanes and holidays. He liked to talk about things like that. He doesn't do that any more because he's in heaven now.

Joe
Friend/peer

People on the autism spectrum may require additional support to maintain their relationship with the person who is dying, or to open up a dialogue of remembrance following their death. There exists the same vulnerability in the peer group of the person who is dying that we devalue the strength of their relationships with others. Social communciation and understanding difficulties may make people on the autism spectrum express themselves and form relationships in a way that doesn't conform to social norms.

As challenging an experience as the palliative care and death of a peer or housemate may be for someone on the autism spectrum, it also creates a valuable opportunity for learning; facilitating discussion about difficult subject matter in an appropriate and meaningful context. Faherty (2008) encourages practitioners to educate individuals with autism about self-knowledge and to view bereavement as an opportunity to build strength from experience.

> *"The ultimate aims of staff should be to enable clients not only to achieve a successful resolution of grief, but also to enable them to transform their experience into a source of strength…"*
>
> (Allison, 1992)

Family and friends

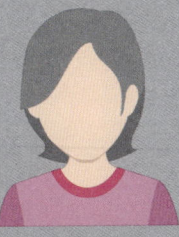

Marian
Mum

> Stephane had a very sensitive side and he could sense when his mum was worried or unhappy. He knew.

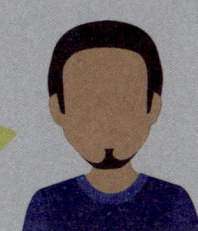

Justin
Support worker

> We were fortunate we had a good relationship with Stephane's mother, that was important and it grew stronger as we cared for him towards the end. But to see her watching her son die, that was hard for us to watch.

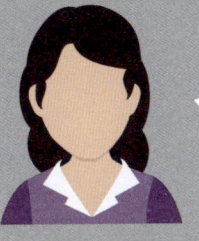

Kirsty
Keyworker

> We would phone his mum as often as we could to keep her up to date, tell her if he'd had a good or a bad day. She would come down from Aberdeen as often as she could and sit with him. We took Stephane up to see his mother and the whole family came together for a family meal. And for us as outsiders to that family looking in it was difficult. We were seeing a family about to lose someone they loved, and whom we cared for too. You can't go through something like that with a family and not think about them for ever more.

The holistic nature of palliative and end of life care often involves a degree of support for the other significant people in the person's life too. We need to acknowledge the importance of our role in maintaining key relationships for the person on the autism spectrum we are supporting and also recognising elements of shared feelings and experiences of loss between all relevant figures of support and care in that person's life.

Supporting relationships between people on the autism spectrum and their family and friends

> *"We cannot help the terminally ill patient in a really meaningful way if we do not include his family. They play a significant role during the time of illness and their reactions will contribute a lot to the patient's response to… illness."*
>
> (Kubler-Ross, 1973)

One of the vital components of social support as the end of a person's life approaches will be in ensuring that the person on the autism spectrum and those closest to them have opportunities to form final memories and shared experiences together. Ensuring there are opportunities for shared time together could be invaluable for people on the autism spectrum who may struggle to initiate social contact and events themselves and for family members who recognise that quality time together is now time limited as a result of the person's prognosis.

People on the autism spectrum who thrive on predictability in their relationships and struggle with aspects of social understanding may require additional support or preparation to understand the qualitatively differing interactions that may arise with those who love them. The people who are important to them in their lives may be struggling with their own feelings and emotions, or the nature of their interactions and roles may differ because of the limited nature of their time together.

It has been highlighted in a 2013 report by Autism Europe on the rights of ageing people with autism that the parents of an adult on the autism spectrum will also be facing their own health and age-related issues and support and accommodations may be required to help them maintain relationships with their son or daughter that recognise their own particular challenges or life circumstances (Baranger and Sullings, 2013). This will be particularly felt for families where ageing parents are still primary caregivers. Where this is the case additional support may be required from care services, a carer's assessment to establish the needs of the family, or support from a local carers centre.

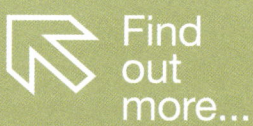

Find out more…

The Carers Trust provides support and advice to carers in Scotland, Wales and Northern Ireland. Where staff, families and friends are acting as primary carers the trust can direct them to sources of support, advice and local services.

www.carers.org

Relationships between care staff and families

It is possible that family members may seek support from care staff because they have known and understood the person who is dying in a way that few other people in the life of the person potentially have. As a result of their understanding and feelings towards the person they are supporting, care staff could be considered particularly qualified to lend an ear to families who need to talk (Allison, 2001).

Families may want to reminisce about the past, they may express extremes of emotion. They may be looking for care staff to share their own memories or experiences, or require them to take the role of an active listener whose role in the conversation is to listen and reflect back that they have understood what has been expressed. Sometimes the support might take the form of being comfortable sitting in silence and respecting the need for quiet time and reflection. Some families will view the care teams as professionals, their interactions with whom are confined to sharing of information. In some cases families would view particular types of questioning or conversation as intrusive.

There also exists a potential for miscommunication and differing opinions between families and care professionals that could result in conflict or relationship difficulties. It has been established that whatever the differing perspectives of carers and significant people in the person's life, these are often overcome by a mutual desire for truthful communication (Munn et al, 2008). This is important when considering the integrity of what we share and communicate to all relevant parties in conversations about palliative and end of life care. All interactions with significant people in the person's life should be handled with respect and sensitivity and communication channels must be established to ensure that all relevant information regarding a person's care and support is passed on as appropriate to do so. The interactions with providers and experiences of support throughout a person's life will influence a family's future engagement with care teams and social workers (D'Astous et al, 2014). Strong partnerships between care staff and families enable the best possible care for the person through their illness and at the end of their life and this is equally true for their involvement with health services too.

> *"Family and other carers should be involved as a matter of course as partners in the provision of treatment and care, unless good reason is given and Trust Boards should ensure that reasonable adjustments are made to enable them to do this effectively."*
>
> (Mencap, 2007)

Pause for thought...

It is important that care staff read the responses and follow the lead of families and significant people in the person's life so they can adapt their interactions and supports to the needs of each person.

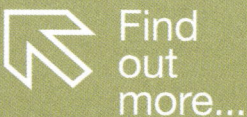

Find out more...

Thinking Ahead
A Planning Guide for Families

Thinking Ahead is a resource designed to enable families to make person centred plans for the future. It has been developed with the intention of providing a framework for families who fear they will not be around to advocate for their family members in the future at times of significant life events and transitions. It also provides useful guidance and discussion points around future planning and acts as a tool to enable families to express their wishes and aspirations.

Foundation for People with Learning Disabilities

www.learningdisabilities.org.uk

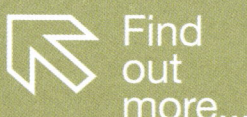

Find out more...

Partnership Working with Family Carers of People with a Learning Disability and People with Autism

This book written by a family carer and colleague describes the contribution that many family carers make to the lives of people with a learning disability and people with autism. It explains how support workers can work well in partnership with family carers.

BILD

www.bild.org.uk/books

To aid effective communication and partnership working, it is worthwhile to put in place protocols with families establishing what people's expectations are regarding:

- what information is passed on
- by what means
- by whom
- under what circumstances and how often

Protocols should factor in the needs and wishes of the person with the life-limiting illness around sharing of personal information. Where a person or persons have legal authority to be involved in decision making and overseeing the welfare of the person on the autism spectrum communication protocols must also reflect this.

Peaceful, Pain Free and Dignified

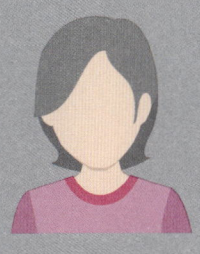

Marian
Mum

I was kept well informed and that was important. I take my hat off to the wonderful people who kept me so well informed. I came down as often as I could to see Stephane and I got great support from the staff. It was more difficult for my other children who didn't live nearby.

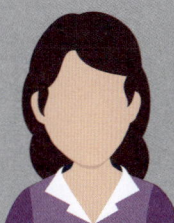

Kirsty
Keyworker

There were some times when news was better coming from Stephane's sister to his mother than coming directly from the support staff, because she knew her mum best. When Stephane passed away thankfully his mum was there, and I think she felt comfortable with us because she knew us well. It wasn't like she was a stranger sitting here, she was in her son's house and that's how it should have been. We would just sit with her and listen. I think that was one of the most important ways we could offer our support to her, by just listening to her. She wanted to talk, to talk about when Stephane was young, to talk about the family, and we just listened.

Depending on the relationship between support services and families and the personal needs and wishes of those closest to the person who has died, it may be appropriate to maintain some form of contact with families following the person's death in the interests of ongoing support and sensitivity to the family's loss. This might be in the form of a letter, a phone call, or a card that acknowledges the loss and sends a message that the loss of the person they have both known and supported has not been forgotten. For some families breaking contact with the support service may be part of the process of gaining closure on the person's death. For others whose family member has been in long-term care of that service it might be comforting to have acknowledgment that the service has been a longstanding part of their life as well as that of their family member.

In *Caring for People with Learning Disabilities who are Dying* Noelle Blackman highlights the issue of ongoing contact between support services and family after the death of the person.

> *"All too often, families say that once their relative with a learning disability had died, the service world forgets them. It would be comforting for many families to know they had not been forgotten."*
>
> (Blackman and Todd, 2005)

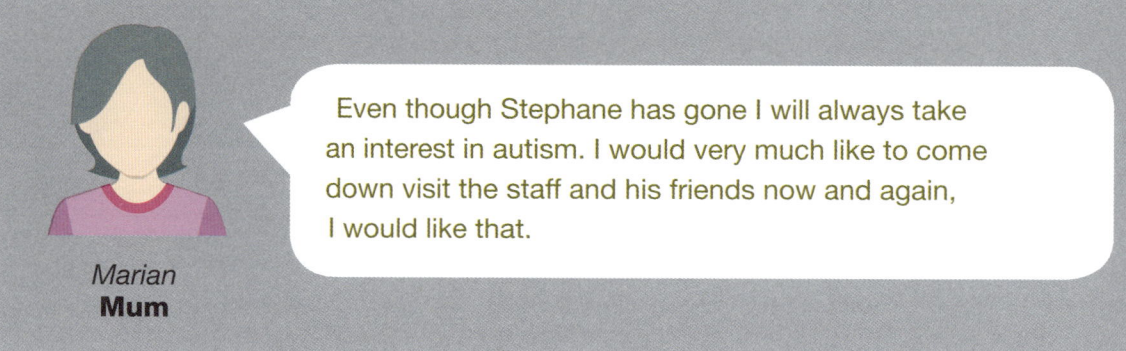

Marian
Mum

Even though Stephane has gone I will always take an interest in autism. I would very much like to come down visit the staff and his friends now and again, I would like that.

Support from other agencies

Social support is often classified in terms of someone *"getting their affairs in order"* (Department of Health, 2006). Exploration of terms such as 'social support' may be complicated by the correlation between a diagnosis of autism and social communication and understanding issues. However, there will also be practical and administrative support required managing practical challenges in someone's support and care that will influence relationships between social care staff and other professionals.

Social work

For individuals who are not in 24-hour care, social workers may be able to commission services for people on the autism spectrum to help them with practical aspects of day-to-day living that they are no longer able to take part in. They may also be able to put in additional referrals and provide sources of support for the person with a life-limiting illness and their carers.

There may be a requirement for higher ratios of staff support in care services that need to be negotiated with social work teams to secure an appropriate level of support and funding for the person on the autism spectrum at the end of their life.

Finance and benefits

The person's entitlement to benefits such as their PIP (personal independence payment) may be affected by the diagnosis of a life-limiting illness for someone not already in receipt of higher rates of entitlement. Your social worker can tell you more about entitlements, or you can get more information from the Department of Work and Pensions (www.gov.uk/browse/benefits).

Advocacy

There might be the need to involve an independent advocate to ensure that the person on the autism spectrum remains at the heart of all decisions affecting their care and treatment. This could be of particular value where there are conflicting views on a person's care, in the event of a need to challenge a decision, or when the person has no family to advocate on their behalf.

> **Pause for thought...**
>
> Social workers and care managers should be alerted as soon as possible to the changing care needs of the person diagnosed with a life-limiting illness to ensure responsiveness of support.

Support for care staff

When looking at issues of loss and bereavement it has been theorised that there often exists a correlation between an individual's management of their grief and the experience and understanding of their support workers (McKechnie, 2006). It therefore follows that particular attention is required to ensure that care staff feel confident, able and well-informed to support people on the autism spectrum, their peers and families, in the event of a diagnosis of life-limiting illness through to the person's death.

Social care services must anticipate the grief reactions of staff, particularly those who have developed close support relationships with the person on the autism spectrum and possibly over a long period of time. The nature of their support for someone at such a significant moment in their life can be both enriching and distressing (Wright, 2007). In a 2014 study exploring grief after patient death for care staff, researchers concluded that symptoms of grief similar to those experienced by family carers were common amongst direct care workers (Boerner et al, 2015).

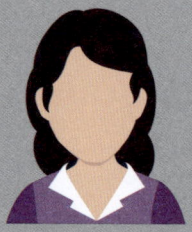

Kirsty
Keyworker

> Even though you're there as a paid carer, a professional, the most difficult thing when you've known and supported someone for a length of time is to not let your emotions take over. That's not saying you should ignore your feelings. It was important that the team could talk to each other and be honest about how we felt. But you want to do the best you can and the best we could do for Stephane was to be professional. And in circumstances like those you want to do your best.

A lack of support for carers, which is likely to be true for both paid and unpaid carers, is considered one of the main contributing factors to situations where the person with a life-limiting illness is no longer able to stay in their own homes following what has been described as a *"crisis led"* approach to support and care planning (Thomas, 2006). Ensuring support staff feel equipped to do their job in these difficult circumstances is also essential to avoid high turnover of care staff. This includes opportunities to take a step back from the intensity of the situation, find opportunities for relaxation and time to support each other (Wright, 2007).

> *"Just as we have to breathe in and breathe out, people have to 'recharge their batteries' outside the sickroom at times, live a normal life from time to time; we cannot function efficiently in the constant awareness of the illness."*
>
> (Kubler-Ross, 1973)

Continuity of support is imperative as changes in staffing can be intrusive and difficult to cope with (Beresford et al, 2007), particularly for a service user group who may experience challenges building relationships of trust with key support figures in their life. The distress caused by changes in formal caregivers has also been linked to poorer health outcomes for individuals dependent on support from carers (Winkler et al, 2011).

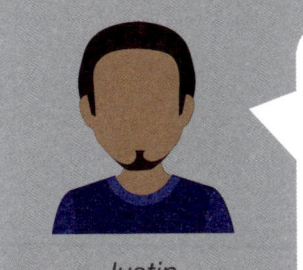

Justin
Support worker

"In the last months of Stephane's life it was the same core team supporting him and that was important. We knew him, we knew his medication, we knew how to look for signs that he was in pain or uncomfortable. If I could pass on one message to other care staff it would be the importance of that staff team consistency at the end of the person's life."

For staff teams working with individuals on the autism spectrum, often the people we know and support encourage us to challenge our own views and outlooks on life (Isanon, 2008). The diversity of thinking amongst individuals on the autism spectrum on aspects of life and death and relationships prepares social care teams for some of the difficult conversations and differing viewpoints they are used to managing, embracing and resolving with the people they know and support.

The trust that emerges between the person on the autism spectrum and a member of support staff who has taken time throughout the person's life to acknowledge their viewpoint and respect their individuality builds support relationships conducive to open dialogue and sensitive care from diagnosis through to the end of the person's life. Social support following a diagnosis of life-limiting illness should be delivered by those people who can reaffirm the person's individuality and self identity and appreciate what and who matters to them in their life.

Social: final thoughts

In her 2003 publication *Loss and Learning Disability* Noelle Blackman includes a model for assessing grief responses for a person with learning disabilities. Whilst designed for those individuals with a learning disability, the model provides a framework of thoughts and questions that are of relevance to people on the autism spectrum without additional learning disabilities and indeed for those of us not on the autism spectrum going through a period of loss in our lives. The nature of the questions included in the assessment model remind us of both the fundamental commonalities of grief responses in us all, and also the individuality of response across people regardless of diagnoses or perceived levels of ability. The model recognises that issues of ageing, illness, death and grief are universal and fundamental to our sense of being and interrelatedness.

Bereavement and loss of any nature has been described as *"the state of being caught between the present, a past and a lost future"* (Walter, 1999). It may then be important for people who know the person well and have shared in significant moments in their life to put thought and effort into helping them construct a personal biography of their life as they approach their death.

Significant moments need not only be about the seemingly big moments and conversations as someone approaches the end of their life. The National Council for Palliative Care published a document called *Small is Beautiful* in 2010 that recognised:

> *"we're told time and again that it's the small things that make a difference. We wanted to remind providers and commissioners that they don't have to change the world to provide responsive care – they can change care here and now in the small, thoughtful things that they do."*

(National Council for Palliative Care, 2010)

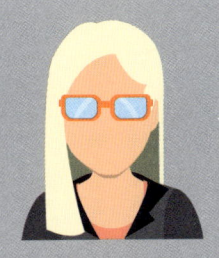

Valerie
Manager

Euan was kind to Stephane and would ask him how he was feeling every day. Sometimes he would call on staff if he thought Stephane needed support, and he would buy him a magazine if he was out.

The writer Damian Milton writes of his feelings that people on the autism spectrum are "*often deeply misunderstood and stigmatized in a society unforgiving to the needs of autistic people*" (Milton, 2014).

In autism support services we tend to focus on the differences between us and the people on the autism spectrum we support. This is not with the intention of creating social divides, but rather with the intention of developing an understanding of their individual viewpoint and thinking style thus enabling a person centred approach to care that embraces the diversity of people diagnosed as being on the autism spectrum.

The tension that exists between understanding our similarities and embracing differences between people on the autism spectrum and those who are not will always feel particularly profound when looking at issues of social support and relationships. Social support during palliative and end of life care must encompass that developed understanding of the relationships and connections between the person on the autism spectrum and all those involved in their life and care.

Social

Discussion points for care teams

- People are often fearful about communicating issues of end of life care with the individuals on the autism spectrum they know and support, their families, friends and peers. What aspects would you personally find challenging and why?

- How perceptive is the person on the autism spectrum you know/support to the emotional and stress responses of those around them?

- People diagnosed with a life-limiting illness are often highlighted as being at risk of becoming socially isolated as their illness progresses. How would you support the people on the autism spectrum you know/support to maintain important relationships? Might the social expectations of family and friends differ to those of the person with autism?

- Consistency of staffing was cited by the care team as key to the success of Stephane's palliative care. Why do you think this was so important?

Social: support mapping for care teams

People diagnosed with a life-limiting illness are cited as vulnerable to loss of social relationships and networks as their ability to form and sustain social relationships can be challenged by the complexities of their autism, it is important to consider how they will maintain and in some cases redefine the relationships and interactions they have with the significant people within their life.

Carers Trust provides support and advice to staff, families and friends with caring responsibilities

'Thinking Ahead': a planning guide for families' could be helpful

To aid effective communication and partnership working, we need to put in place protocols with staff, families and friends establishing what people's expectations are regarding:
- what information is passed on
- by what means
- by whom
- under what circumstances and how often

People are often fearful about communicating issues of end of life care with the person on the autism spectrum they support, their families, friends and peers. What aspects of palliative care would you personally find challenging to discuss and why?

How will you ensure consistency and continuity of staffing support? Why do you think this is important?

How can we support families and important people in the individual's life to get involved in planning for the future?

Protocols for communication and sharing of information
- Ahead of hospital visit ensure that hospital passport is available and seek support from LD liaison nurse
- Daily completion of communication book and pain assessment recordings for sharing with community nurses
- Electronic palliative care summary will be updated daily by health/GP
- Medication protocols in place

Protocols for communication and sharing of information
- See protocol in support plan for contact with mum and key family members (detailing what to share and when)
- Reassess arrangements with family as illness progresses.
- Relating to, in event of death, information about his day, passing on information from GP and nurses, documenting family wishes, capturing feedback from the family that informs care and support

How can we support better relationships with health?
- Invite key individuals to team meetings.
- Use of communication diary, pain assessment recordings and hospital passport for sharing important information.
- Link with learning disability liaison nurse for hospital consultations.
- Contacts list in place and accessible to support team at all times.

How can we support the person to maintain important family relationships?
- Respect and listen to family views and wishes
- Spend time looking at family photographs (add to life story book)
- Support for mum to arrange overnight stays locally/family meal
- Family time to be built around usual patterns of contact and activities to maintain familiar routines

What support is required for the care team?
- Consistency of core staff team to ensure effective knowledge sharing and consistency of support for Stephane
- Regular team meetings and opportunities for peer support
- Opportunities to ask questions to health teams/ 24 hour contact information
- Regular 1:1 supervision with manager
- Availability of external counselling services should they be required

Are there supports or strategies required to strengthen relationships?
- Request for meeting with social work to review current level of support and plan for future support needs.
- More frequent review of service required (anticipate support changes and funding implications).

Protocols for communication and sharing of information
- 3 monthly service review meetings
- Update reports to be sent to Elaine via secure email address
- Information to be sent to Lewis to inform updates to social story and visual communication systems

How can we support the person to maintain important relationships with friends and peers?
- Guided by Stephane's physical health and motivation.
- Gradual reduction of day service hours to try and maintain engagement with peer group.
- New opportunities for shared social experiences and reflection on these, add photos to life story book.

Protocols for communication and sharing of information
- See individual support plans for person specific protocols.
- Increased frequency of keyworker or 'talktime' meetings may be required to explore feelings and understanding with figures of trust
- Consider possibility of peer advocacy and support

"When someone you know has died: people with learning disabilities supporting each other" Is there a role for peer advocacy and support?

Social support networks

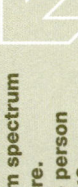

Stephane

Health
Yvonne – Community palliative care nurse
Dr Brodie – GP
Dr McAdam – consultant
Anna – district nurse
Jim – OT

Family
Mum – Marian
Brother, sisters and nephew

Social care team
Valerie – manager
Kirsty – keyworker
Support team – Justin, Alan, Mary, Gemma, Lauren Stewart

Friends and peers
Euan – housemate
Joe – friend
Shona – friend

Other figures of trust and support
Elaine Morrison – social worker
Lewis – speech and language therapist

Social support involves an understanding of the relationships and connections between the person on the autism spectrum and all those involved in their life and care.
Who are the important people in the life of the person on the autism spectrum that you support?

For example community groups, cultural or religious figures of support, advocacy services, social work, counselling services

Social: support mapping for care teams

People diagnosed with a life-limiting illness are cited as vulnerable to loss of social relationships and networks as their illness progresses. For people on the autism spectrum whose ability to form and sustain social relationships can be challenged by the complexities of their autism, it is important to consider how they will maintain and in some cases redefine the relationships and interactions they have with the significant people within their life.

Carers Trust provides support and advice to staff, families and friends with caring responsibilities

'Thinking Ahead': a planning guide for families' could be helpful

To aid effective communication and partnership working, we need to put in place protocols with staff, families and friends establishing what people's expectations are regarding:
- what information is passed on
- by what means
- by whom
- under what circumstances and how often

People are often fearful about communicating issues of end of life care with the person on the autism spectrum they support, their families, friends and peers. What aspects of palliative care would you personally find challenging to discuss and why?

How will you ensure consistency and continuity of staffing support? Why do you think this is important?

How can we support families and important people in the individual's life to get involved in planning for the future?

What support is required for the care team?

Protocols for communication and sharing of information

How can we support the person to maintain important relationships with friends and peers?

Protocols for communication and sharing of information

How can we support the person to maintain important family relationships?

Protocols for communication and sharing of information

How can we support better relationships with health?

Protocols for communication and sharing of information

Are there supports or strategies required to strengthen relationships?

Protocols for communication and sharing of information

Social support networks

- Social care team
- Friends and peers
- Family
- Health
- Other figures of trust and support

Name

Social support involves an understanding of the relationships and connections between the person on the autism spectrum and all those involved in their life and care.
Who are the important people in the life of the person on the autism spectrum that you support?

For example community groups, cultural or religious figures of support, advocacy services, social work, counselling services

'When someone you know has died: people with learning disabilities supporting each other' Is there a role for peer advocacy and support?

Chapter 4:
Spiritual

Spiritual themes and considerations often come to the fore in discussions about end of life care with an importance and immediacy unsurpassed by most other life events. Spirituality is something that is deeply personal and not easy to define, which will make it particularly difficult to explore with a person on the autism spectrum. Following a diagnosis of a life-limiting illness it is natural, and for many people imperative, to consider themes such as personal meaning, culture, religion and self in the context of their own life and their relationship to the world around them.

Stephane's story

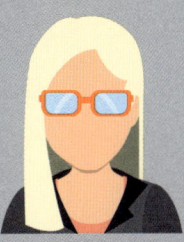

Valerie
Manager

We discussed how we were going to tell Stephane, how we would broach this with him without really knowing what his understanding was going to be. We wanted to know what his hopes would be, what his wishes would be, but it was very difficult because we also didn't want to frighten him.

We spoke to his family, and we had to respect their wishes of course. They decided to tell Stephane he was going to be with Jesus, as his mum felt that he would understand this because when dad passed away that's what they had all been told.

It was sad to see him fading and becoming so thin, I reached a point where I felt it was time for him to pass away. Because right now I know he's at peace in heaven and he's enjoying seeing his father.

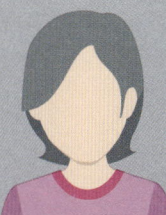

Marian
Mum

Pause for thought...

What implications does this have for the spiritual wellbeing of a person on the autism spectrum from diagnosis of a life-limiting illness through to the end of their life?

We often base our support and assumptions about people on the autism spectrum on spoken words and observable behaviours taken at face value, particularly if we find it hard to relate to or understand the personal beliefs and motivations of the person we are supporting. Spirituality is a very personal and highly subjective area of support. However, at the end of life it is of particular importance to consider spiritual wellbeing and significance for the individuals we are supporting as the consequences of their prognosis could result in the additional distress of a personal crisis of meaning (Swinton, 2006) without sensitive consideration of life meaning, personal beliefs, and religious and cultural practices.

We asked support staff working in autism services what some of the challenges were for the individuals on the autism spectrum they know and support. The challenges most commonly cited were:

- the religious and cultural expectations of others may not be reflective of the person's own beliefs or understanding
- the person may have their own interpretation of spiritual beliefs
- social communication difficulties may affect someone's ability to articulate or express what is meaningful and significant in their life
- what is meaningful and important in the person's life may differ to what those supporting them typically expect
- the prevalence of abstract concepts and terminology when exploring spiritual views and beliefs
- difficulty with reflection on life experiences and definition of self in relation to past events and experiences
- executive functioning issues around planning for the future
- spiritual wellbeing and definitions are highly personal and subjective
- a general lack of exploration and acknowledgment of the themes relating to spirituality and personal meaning in the lives of people on the autism spectrum

The search for meaning and significance in life

"There is a growing shared understanding that 'meaning making' and 'life review' are important spiritual processes which can manifest themselves in a variety of ways."

Mowat and O'Neill (2013)

The difficulty that individuals on the autism spectrum may have in expressing what is meaningful within their lives to others leaves them vulnerable to a perception that they lack spiritual beliefs. In her book *Autism and Spirituality* (2013) Olga Bogdashina writes of her concerns about the denial of the spirituality of people on the autism spectrum. She writes of how an interpreted lack of social relatedness to others means we overlook a person's connections to others and their environment and that our readiness to interpret what we see with what someone feels or experiences can hinder a developed understanding of the personal spirituality of people on the autism spectrum.

Religious beliefs

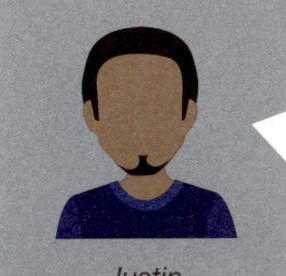

Justin
Support worker

Stephane's family found comfort through their belief in god and heaven. It was hard for us to know Stephane's particular views of religion, and whether or not his family's beliefs were also beliefs he shared. But we recognised that the church had been a part of his life as he was growing up, and an important part of family life. We wanted him to have opportunities to attend church with his family and hoped he may have found comfort in that. Whether that was comfort through faith or through familiarity we didn't know but we hoped it was a place of peace for him in life and in death.

Sundays were always a happy day for Stephane. He had grown up seeing pictures of Jesus and I would read him bible stories. So I explained to him that wonderful things awaited him in heaven and told him that Jesus would look after him. I think this gave him great peace.

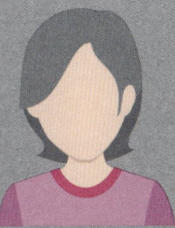

Marian
Mum

Chapter 4: **Spiritual**

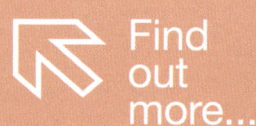

Find out more...

Religious Expression: A Fundamental Human Right

The report of an action research project on meeting the religious needs of people with learning disabilities.

Foundation for People with Learning Disabilities

www.learning disabilities.org.uk

Spirituality is often, but not always, closely linked to religious beliefs and customs and attitudes towards palliative care are often influenced by those beliefs (Steinberg, 2011). It is always important to understand and respect the religious and cultural values and customs of the person you are supporting. Their beliefs can be used positively to help provide explanations and support spiritual wellbeing at an otherwise difficult time. When providing day-to-day support to a person with specific ethnic or religious needs staff need to have an understanding of any daily routines, dietary requirements and personal care needs influenced by their cultural or religious background. After the diagnosis of a life-limiting illness these understandings need to be extended to reflect the issues relating to their new situation.

In their 2004 report *Religious Expression: A Fundamental Human Right* Hatton and colleagues express concern about the lack of supports for people with a learning disability, and therefore a significant percentage of people on the autism spectrum, to explore and practice religious and spiritual beliefs. They also recognise the potentially positive impact of religious connectedness on the physical and mental health of an individual and their family or support network (Hatton, 2004).

Pause for thought...

If support staff feel that their knowledge of the cultural and religious customs practised by the person or their family is insufficient, it is important to seek advice to ensure a consistent and informed support approach that is respectful of people's beliefs.

Support staff could ask the person they support, their family and friends or local cultural and religious leaders, such as a priest, rabbi, or imam, for further information. Good person centred support should recognise that there are big differences in how people understand and express their faith. The cultural and religious traditions of the person and their family should be respected and observed.

"People of all backgrounds and beliefs may experience spiritual pain and existential crises towards the end of life… staff need to be able to recognise such crises and be aware of how to seek help from representatives of the range of faiths and beliefs in society."

(Davies and Higginson, 2004)

People on the autism spectrum may have differing interpretations of or relationships with religion. Some individuals may find the rhythm and predictability of religious services or meetings helpful. Others may not cope with or be motivated by the collective and institutional nature of conventional religion and so find the need to construct their own spirituality that may still be founded in elements of religious experience and thought (Isanon, 2008; Caldwell-Harris et al, 2011). Whatever the individual's relationship with their religion, it can be positively used to support coping and find peace at a time of loss and possible spiritual distress.

Spiritual understanding and experience

Spiritual beliefs can be difficult to explain and are open to differing interpretations. Sometimes these can be used to provide comfort or explain issues relating to the end of life, but for those individuals who tend to understand things in a very literal way or thrive on concrete means of communication to support their understanding, the abstract nature of the language of spirituality could be difficult to comprehend. People on the autism spectrum may require additional support to make sense of some of the language and terminology of end of life care and the spiritual beliefs and expressions of significant others in their life.

However, it could equally be argued that the language used when exploring spiritual themes at the end of life is often broad and open to interpretation to allow room for people to find their own personal definitions and meanings within those terms. This enables recognition of individual response to spirituality and to the news of life-limiting illness and death.

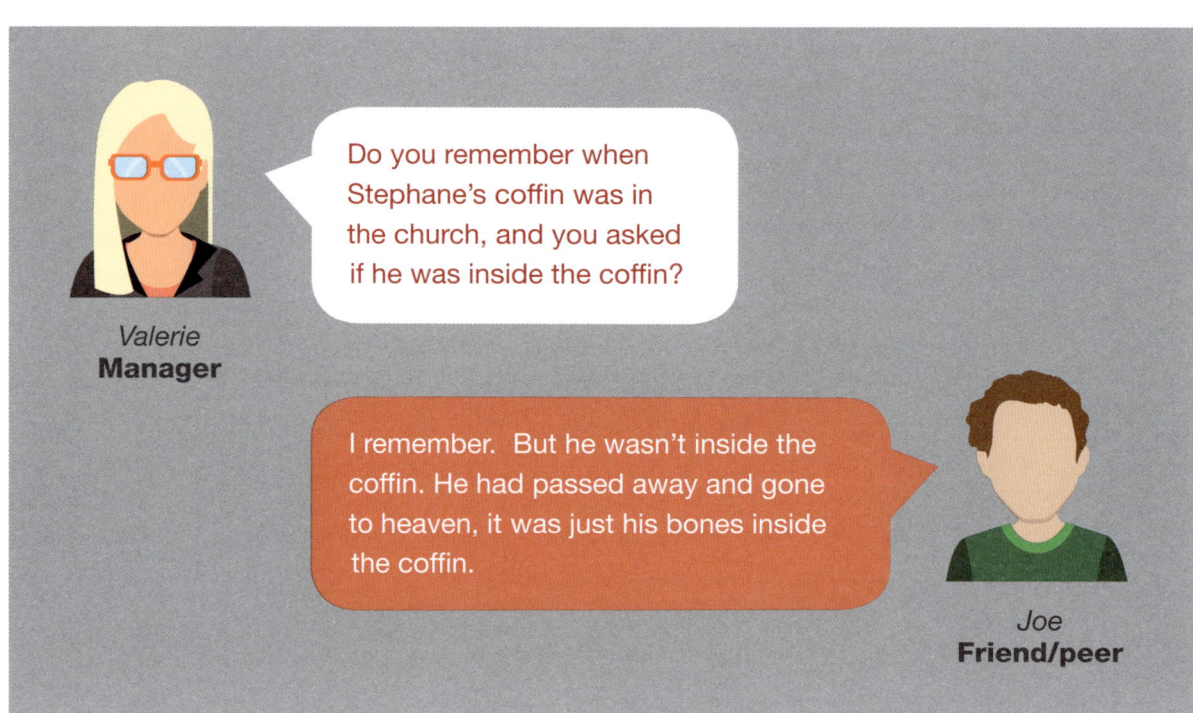

In *Understanding Death and Illness and What they Teach About Life* Catherine Faherty acknowledges the varying beliefs around what happens to someone after they have died:

> *"Do they live on in the memories of others? Is it the end of the person forever? Does the person's soul separate from the shell of their body? Does the life energy of the person live on in another form? Is there some form of 'afterlife'?"*

(Faherty, 2008)

It may be helpful to break questions and topics down to fully explore aspects of someone's beliefs and perceptions.

It is important not to confuse issues relating to understanding of spiritual terminology and communication with spiritual *experience*. The language and comprehension challenges relating to understanding of abstract concepts and broad spiritual themes do not mean that a person lacks spirituality at a level of feeling and experience. It may just be that the means to interpret, make sense of, or communicate issues of spirituality are complicated by aspects of the person's autism. Rita Jordan reminds us that for individuals on the autism spectrum who also have severe learning difficulties language is often a contextual occurrence as opposed to carrying real meaning (Jordan, 2001). Spirituality is about personal meaning and experience and issues relating to language and communication do not exclude people on the autism spectrum from potentially having a deeply felt and profound sense of spirituality.

It has been proposed that differing sensory perceptual experiences of the world predispose people on the autism spectrum to novel existential experiences that support an acute sense of spiritual being (Bogdashina, 2013).

A purposeful understanding of spirituality recognises it is about what we feel and experience, it is not a thing we can hold or a word to be defined. Spirituality is fundamentally human (Isanon, 2008; Hatton et al, 2004) and therefore person centred in the truest sense of the term. Where faith, beliefs and personal experiences differ there is room for acceptance of that diversity of viewpoints in a profound and deeply human way when addressing themes of spirituality for people on the autism spectrum.

Selfhood

One of the most important ways of reflecting on personal meaning in life is to reflect on your knowledge, experiences, memories and relationship to others and your environment; the context of your existence and your understanding of your 'self'.

The origins of the word 'autism' are rooted in the idea of self and issues of selfhood and self in relation to others. Whilst there is an inherent focus on issues of relationships to others in support services for people on the autism spectrum, with impairments in social understanding and reciprocity cited in the diagnostic criteria for autism spectrum conditions (American Psychiatric Association, 2013; World Health Organisation, 2015a), there is perhaps not always the same focus on understanding the individual's own understanding of self.

Similarly to unpicking the term spiritual, to understand what we mean by the term self involves what the neuroscientist VS Ramachandran considers *"a lumping together of many different phenomena"*. He identifies five key characteristics of self to help us understand the complexity of defining self (Ramachandran, 2003):

- **Continuity of self**, in relation to past, present and future
- **Unity of self**, bringing all our experiences, thoughts and beliefs into one self
- **Ownership of self**, feeling anchored in your own body
- **Agency of self**, free will to be in charge of your own destiny
- **Reflection on self**, awareness

Pause for thought...

For people on the autism spectrum who struggle to place themselves in the context of their life narrative, support may be required to help them map out what and who has been important in their lives to strengthen their sense of self identity and personal meaning as they approach the end of their life.

Rita Jordan writes of impairment of self awareness in people on the autism spectrum who have learning disabilities (Jordan, 2001) and Damien Milton writes of the challenges of understanding self in relation to autobiographical memory, describing memories as *"not placed into a continuous narrative of selfhood with any ease"* (Milton, 2014). It could therefore be proposed that there are challenges for individuals on the autism spectrum in having a fully developed sense of self when we compare their experiences to Ramachandran's criteria of self. This does not mean that the person lacks selfhood but their sense of self-identity may be qualitatively different, fragmented, underdeveloped in one of those key areas, or they may have difficulty experiencing a sense of self (Bogdashina, 2013).

Encouraging the person you are supporting to create a life story book is a useful way of helping them reflect on what is meaningful in their life.

- Life story can be captured in a range of different media. It might be important to use a range of formats or multi-sensory tools to engage and evoke memories or a sense of time and place. In addition to use of images and written word it might be useful to include tangible objects of reference, audio, scents, textures or video, or create a memory box (Towers, 2013).

- Life story doesn't need to be explored chronologically, let the person you are supporting decide where they are comfortable starting (Blackman, 2003). Some individuals will benefit from dividing their life story book into clearly defined life themes or chronological order to offer them direction and make it easier to initiate discussion. A less ordered and more expressive approach to reflection may work for other individuals, particularly if it is more in keeping with their perception of self. They may be more comfortable with *"a sense of self that is fragmented or 'nomadic' in nature"* (Milton, 2014).

- Use of a loose leaf format means that the book can continually be added to and the sequence is flexible (Blackman, 2003).

The strategies for reflection on life stories and relationships used in the creation of life story books will be equally applicable when providing support for the peer group of the person with life-limiting illness as the person they know and share their life with approaches the end of their life and dies. One of the determinants of *"successful grieving"* is the integration of the deceased person into the life story of the people who live on (Murray Parkes, 1998).

> *"Memories of the deceased serve as an essential bridge between the world with and the world without the loved person"*
>
> (Buchsbaum 1996)

A person going through a process of life-limiting illness will typically expect to see physical changes to their body and may experience an altered sense of body image as a result of this. Where someone is experiencing self-identity issues related to a loss of self-ability and autonomy, this could be further compounded by changes related to their physical sense of self.

Not addressing such issues in the typical population can have implications for self-esteem, recognition of self and levels of motivation or distress (Wright, 2007). It could be proposed there exists an additional fragility of self-identity in individuals on the autism spectrum who require specialist support from people who know and understand them and the component parts of what constitutes their very individual sense of self to counter loss of psychological wellbeing in this way.

Milberg et al (2014) explored the influencing factors in a patient's sense of security for those with a limited life expectancy. Self-efficacy and maintaining self identity were both highlighted as having a relationship to the person's sense of security and wellbeing during the process of palliative care (Milberg et al, 2014). Gunilla Gerland writes of the importance of promoting self esteem and efficacy for people on the autism spectrum in relation to the power balance that exists between the individual and the people who care for them (Gerland, 2013). The sense of powerlessness to affect the decisions and outcomes in their life may be profoundly felt for a person on the autism spectrum following a diagnosis of life-limiting illness and throughout the ensuing care, where both health and social care staff take decisions regarding their care and their ability to self advocate may be further compromised by the acute nature of their illness.

> "As I grew to accept that being different is a natural part of the human condition, I felt less compelled to hide the parts of me that openly identify me as different. I began to reclaim and take ownership of my autistic traits."
> (Kim, 2014)

Following diagnosis, issues of self are at the fore of the process of life reflection and finding an inner peace linked to spiritual wellbeing. People on the autism spectrum may require support to take ownership of their identity or place themselves in the context of their lives, thus finding acceptance based on their own unique sense of spiritual awareness. Understanding of spirituality begins with the self and explores what and who is important in that person's life.

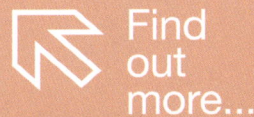 Find out more...

What If:

Celebrating My Life

NHS North East Lincolnshire

This is a document designed to enable people to set out their wishes for how they would like their care to be delivered in their final days in a way that recognises what is important to them in their life. It helps the person retain a sense of self control over what will happen to them at the end of their life.

www.pcpld.com

Religious and cultural customs

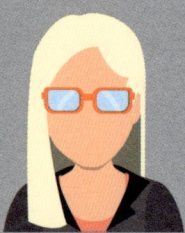

Valerie
Manager

Planning his funeral we wanted to know what Stephane's wishes were but that was challenging with his comprehension and communication difficulties. We thought how on earth will we use a communication board or a script to say 'cremation or burial'?

But following on from this experience, his peers on the autism spectrum who live here and have shared Stephane's life with him were able to attend his funeral. And a couple of them have been able to voice that they would prefer to be buried. So it's helped them, and helped us supporting them, to open up a discussion about their wishes should something happen to them.

When he passed away Stephane was cremated not buried. When my time comes I would like to be buried instead of cremated because I would feel safer being buried.

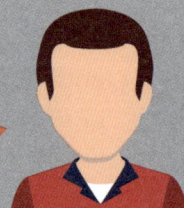

Euan
Housemate

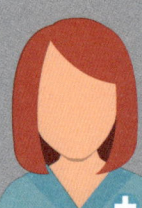

Yvonne
Nurse

We all know from an early age that we're going to die but we never want to discuss it, and that's if we don't have any kind of learning difficulty or communication challenge. So for someone with autism to be able to voice that it's fantastic. There's been a real cohesion of learning for all concerned. For the other individuals living here to want their support staff to know what their wishes are is really good to hear.

Peaceful, Pain Free and Dignified

The religious and cultural beliefs and practices of the person and their family are important to understand as part of our responsibility to provide good person centred support. This is particularly important when planning end of life care. This may have implications for how the person is treated before the end of their life, immediately after they die and the ceremonial goodbyes following their death.

For example:

- Is there the requirement for the attendance of a priest, imam or other spiritual leader?
- Should the coffin be open or closed?
- Do specific items need to be placed within the coffin?
- Are there specific words and prayers that need to be said?
- Are there special requirements for the preparation of the body?
- Are there timeframes for particular events and rituals?
- What implications do beliefs about after life have for customs and ceremonies?
- If support teams don't feel they have a developed understanding of the cultural or religious needs of the person they are supporting it is important to seek advice. In some religions and cultures there will be very specific rituals and expectations about what must happen following someone's death.
- For other people there will be an emphasis on personalisation of rituals and ceremonies to celebrate the life of the person who has died, recognising and expressing their individuality.

Saying goodbye

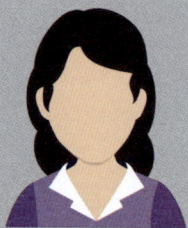

Kirsty **Keyworker**

> At the funeral it was very emotional when they took the coffin away. A couple of Stephane's friends who were also on the autism spectrum turned and waved and said goodbye to Stephane. We had told them we were going to pay our respects and to say goodbye, and that's what they were doing, saying goodbye.

"After the storm passed, I stayed beneath the table. It took me the rest of the day before I would venture out. I think this was the case, because I was surprised the storm was over. It was hard to trust that it had really gone – I mean, how can something be there for a moment or longer and then not there anymore?"

(Lawson, 2000)

The opportunity to attend the funeral of the deceased may be an important opportunity to 'experience' the bereavement and find closure on their loss for a person on the autism spectrum. Physical participation in a ceremony designed both to say goodbye (reinforcing the finality of death) and often establish rituals that can be repeated as a way of developing an ongoing relationship with the deceased (such as visiting a gravestone, memorial books and events), can be of great value. Noelle Blackman (Blackman and Todd, 2005) advocates finding ways to promote involvement in funerals and their preparation, such as choosing flowers, saying something at the funeral or contributing plans for the wake.

It has been proposed that there is a fear individuals with learning and communication difficulties are excluded from funerals because of a presumed inability to cope (Blackman, 2003), or possibly a fear of inappropriate social responses and reactions to a sensitive event. To deny someone the opportunity to attend the funeral or devalue their response to loss in this way could be perceived as dismissive of their grief and perpetuating issues of low self worth.

For other individuals the conventions and collective nature of a funeral may not be sufficient to help them validate their feelings and find the closure they require. In these circumstances those who know the person need to support them to find a more intimate or personalised strategy that helps them say goodbye.

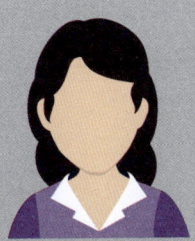

It was important we gave Stephane's flatmates other ways that they could say goodbye. Planting trees, letting go of a helium balloon; we used things we knew had worked previously to help them find closure during times of loss.

Kirsty
Keyworker

Whatever the appropriate way to explore the experience of loss and bereavement for the individuals on the autism spectrum we know and support, experiences like this can provide opportunities to have discussions about life and death in a meaningful context. Learning from life experiences such as this can open up a dialogue about what is of personal significance to the peers on the autism spectrum who have shared in that person's life. This enables support staff to develop a greater understanding of the spiritual needs and wishes of the other people they support and thus prepare them for the future by having a developed understanding of what is meaningful and significant to that person.

Cultural and religious diversity is both celebrated and understood in a multicultural and multi-faith society and it could be proposed we respect and revere the diversity of viewpoints and possibilities this embraces most poignantly and openly when addressing issues of the end of life. Those of us who work in services for people on the autism spectrum can recognise cultures of belief and a collective sense of identity within the communities of people on the autism spectrum we know and support. Therefore we must equally respect and embrace the viewpoints of both the individual and the autism community when looking at issues of spirituality, of meaning in relation to our sense of self and belonging to others and the context of our lives. We have a responsibility to ensure the voices of people who struggle to articulate or express meaning, or whose views and beliefs may differ from conventional 'norms', are not overlooked throughout and at the end of their life.

A good death

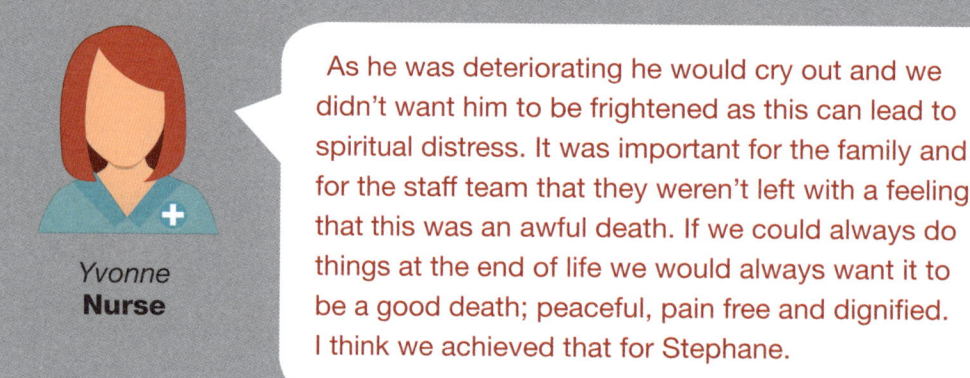

> As he was deteriorating he would cry out and we didn't want him to be frightened as this can lead to spiritual distress. It was important for the family and for the staff team that they weren't left with a feeling that this was an awful death. If we could always do things at the end of life we would always want it to be a good death; peaceful, pain free and dignified. I think we achieved that for Stephane.

Yvonne **Nurse**

'A good death' is a term used by palliative care professionals which at first seems incongruent to the situation. However, the idea of a 'good' death in some ways encompasses the ideas of spiritual wellbeing explored in this section of the practice guide.

Munn et al (2008), reporting research into end of life experiences for individuals in long term care services, identify what they term the components of a 'good death'. They include themes such as dignity, comfort, closure, symptom management, circumstances of death and spiritual belief as determinants of a "*good death*" (Munn et al, 2008).

The necessity for the person at the end of their life and those who they are survived by to feel that at the end of their life the person was as well cared for and as fulfilled as they could be brings a sense of peace that is imperative when considering issues of spiritual wellbeing.

The spirituality of a person on the autism spectrum can give meaning not just to their own life, but also to that of the person supporting them (Isanon, 2008). It is important not just for the person diagnosed with a life-limiting illness, but also to the spiritual wellbeing of those who know and support them throughout their life to feel that they have had a 'good death' so that they are not left with feelings of unresolved distress or regret.

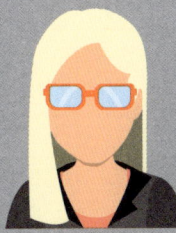

Valerie
Manager

We wanted to help Stephane produce his own bucket list I suppose, for want of a better term.

Yeah I was trying to think of how to phrase it but yes, a bucket list as we would call it. We wanted his final days, months, as it turned out years, to be full of all the things that were important to him in his life. As full of positive experiences and moments that mattered to him as possible.

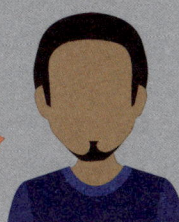

Justin
Support worker

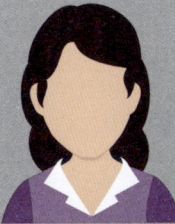

Kirsty
Keyworker

And he needed people who knew him and made him feel safe to do that. I think he did have a good quality of life in his last few years with us, I'm glad looking back I feel we can say that.

Chapter 4: **Spiritual**

Spiritual: final thoughts

"Living in the light of our dying can help us live better now and points to the deeper values and meaning of life itself. If we get it right for the dying, we get it right for the living too."

(Thomas, 2011)

It has been proposed that we all, regardless of autism, communication difficulty, world-view or indeed diagnosis of a life-limiting illness, have difficulty discussing our *"inner worlds"* (Bogdashina, 2013). To define someone based on outward behaviours or the physical symptoms of their illness denies the depth and meaningfulness of the inner reality of people on the autism spectrum that we must endeavour to appreciate when addressing the spiritual needs of the person we are supporting at the end of their life.

Isanon (2008) reminds those who know and support individuals on the autism spectrum that to fail to look beyond the stereotypes and symptoms of a presumed disorder is to fail to value their differing and unique perspectives. The societal creation of social stereotypes and subcultures is based on a need for predictability, simplification and order in life (Hogg and Abrams, 1988). We often reflect on the inflexibility of individuals on the autism spectrum as they take aspects of their life and interactions and put them into metaphorical 'boxes' to help make predictable sense of life. As 'neurotypical' people we often fail to see the boxes that we put other people in to make sense and order of a life open to a breadth of personal and cultural interpretations and spiritual meaning.

Spirituality in essence is a subjective and personal response to the quest for meaning, self-knowing and significance in life. The perceptions and perspectives of the individuals on the autism spectrum we know and support can broaden our own outlooks on spirituality and meaning. We need to take time to understand and embrace differing viewpoints – it could be argued that these are never more fundamental than they are at the end of a person's life.

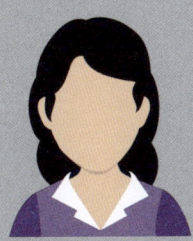

Kirsty
Keyworker

> Joe told me he thinks he might be able to go to heaven and come back down when he wants. I told him that I think when you go to heaven you have to stay there but he told me no that we would both come down together. He said he would ask god, god will say it's OK, we'll hold hands, we'll jump through the clouds, and then we'll go back.
>
> I don't know. I don't know what's in heaven so how can I tell him it's different. And if that gives him some comfort thinking that we can jump through the clouds then so be it.

Pause for thought...

How would you find out about and celebrate the cultural and religious/spiritual background of a person with autism you support?

Spiritual

Discussion points for care teams

- Spiritual themes and ideas often involve quite abstract and difficult to explain concepts. How do we provide literal or meaningful explanations for things that we ourselves find difficult to explain?
For example: **Heaven**

- How would you describe your thoughts on what heaven is to a friend?

- How would you describe heaven to a person on the autism spectrum you know/support?

- Stephane's end of life care opened up a dialogue about death and illness with some of his peers. How can you take difficult experiences and facilitate opportunities for learning and discussions with the people on the autism spectrum you know/support?

Discuss:
Peaceful, pain free and dignified: a good death

Spiritual: support mapping for care teams

Spiritual themes and considerations often come to the fore in discussions about end of life with an importance and immediacy unsurpassed by most other life events. Spirituality is something that is deeply personal and not easy to define which will make it particularly difficult to explore with the person we are supporting on the autism spectrum. Following a diagnosis of a life-limiting illness it is natural, and for many people imperative, to consider themes such as: personal meaning, culture, religion, and self in the context of our own life and our relationship to the world around us.

> Spiritual themes and ideas often involve quite abstract and difficult to define concepts. How do we provide meaningful explanations for things we find difficult to explain?

Religious and cultural customs

What are the important beliefs the person has as a result of their culture or religion?

Stephane has grown up attending church throughout his life with his family who have strong Christian beliefs.

They have explained to him that he is 'going to be with Jesus'

Are there customs, rituals or cultural expectations we must adhere to when considering issues of end of life?

The care team have spoken to Stephane's family about their wishes at the end of his life and plans for his funeral.

These are detailed within his individual support plan.

There will be a Church of Scotland funeral service in the local churches that have been an important part of his life.

If support staff feel that their knowledge of the cultural and religious customs practised by the person or their family is insufficient, it is important to seek advice to ensure a consistent and informed support approach that is respectful of people's beliefs.

> 'Religious Expression: a fundamental human right' could be helpful

Terms and phrases used

'going to be with Jesus'

Understanding of term

It is hard to know Stephane's exact understanding of the term used due to his communication and comprehension difficulties but he accepted this explanation when his father passed away and during previous losses in life (use of terminology linked to prior life experiences)

Strategies to support understanding/alternative means of communicating information

Stephane may point to the sky to indicate 'heaven'

Stephane's mum has tried to explain what heaven may be like to him and that 'Jesus will look after you in heaven'

Stephane's mum has shared pictorial illustrations of Jesus with him using bible stories

> 'Peaceful, pain free and dignified: a good death'
>
> 'What if: celebrating my life' could be helpful

What would a 'good death' be for the person you are supporting?

It would be preferable that Mum is present and there to comfort and support Stephane

Pain free

Free of fear and anxiety in the comfort of his home

That in the time left, Stephane has plenty of opportunities to enjoy things that are important in his life – build positive memories

Who is important in the person's life?

Family is important to Stephane and his Mum in particular.

Stephane's support team

Stephane has been supported by Scottish Autism for many years and is part of an extended community of friends and peers who he has known throughout his life.

What is important in the person's life?

Support from figures of trust – mum and core staff team

Special occasions and celebrations such as Easter

Aeroplanes

Food

Familiarity and routine

Outings and time spent outdoors at favourite places and locations

Looking at magazines and pictures

What are the experiences that have shaped the person's life?

Stephane's father passed away when he was a child. Stephane understands his dad is in heaven with Jesus.

Stephane's time spent in church singing and listening to music and bible stories

Shared memories from his childhood in Scotland and France, family time has been important throughout his life

Does the person require support to place themselves in the context of their life story?

Creation of a life story book with photos and pictures

Opportunities to add to this with photographs documenting new memories and experiences

Support team to spend time with Stephane reflecting on memories and events from his past using the life story book

Creating a life story book could be helpful

Encouraging the person you are supporting to create a life story book is a useful way of helping them reflect on what is meaningful in their life

- You can use a range of media: images, written word, objects, video, audio
- Life story doesn't have to be explored chronologically, be guided by the person.
- Use of a loose leaf format means that the sequence is flexible and can be changed or added to.

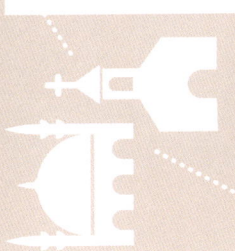

Stephane

Personal meaning in life

Spiritual: support mapping for care teams

Spiritual themes and considerations often come to the fore in discussions about end of life with an importance and immediacy unsurpassed by most other life events. Spirituality is something that is deeply personal and not easy to define which will make it particularly difficult to explore with the person we are supporting on the autism spectrum. Following a diagnosis of a life-limiting illness it is natural, and for many people imperative, to consider themes such as: personal meaning, culture, religion, and self in the context of our own life and our relationship to the world around us.

> Spiritual themes and ideas often involve quite abstract and difficult to define concepts. How do we provide meaningful explanations for things we find difficult to explain?

Religious and cultural customs

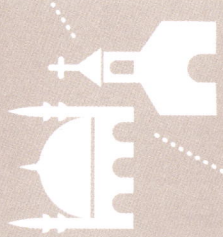

What are the important beliefs the person has as a result of their culture or religion?

Are there customs, rituals or cultural expectations we must adhere to when considering issues of end of life?

If support staff feel that their knowledge of the cultural and religious customs practised by the person or their family is insufficient, it is important to seek advice to ensure a consistent and informed support approach that is respectful of people's beliefs.

> 'Religious Expression: a fundamental human right' could be helpful

Creating a life story book could be helpful

Encouraging the person you are supporting to create a life story book is a useful way of helping them reflect on what is meaningful in their life

- You can use a range of media: images, written word, objects, video, audio
- Life story doesn't have to be explored chronologically, be guided by the person.
- Use of a loose leaf format means that the sequence is flexible and can be changed or added to.

Terms and phrases used

Understanding of term

Strategies to support understanding/alternative means of communicating information

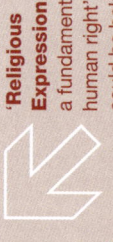

> 'Peaceful, pain free and dignified: a good death'

> 'What if: celebrating my life' could be helpful

What would a 'good death' be for the person you are supporting?

Who is important in the person's life?

What is important in the person's life?

What are the experiences that have shaped the person's life?

Does the person require support to place themselves in the context of their life story?

Name

Personal meaning in life

Perspectives

In our process of exploring themes of palliative and end of life care for people on the autism spectrum over the last two years we have been fortunate to have met and entered into discussion with a range of honest and insightful individuals who have shared their thoughts and views with us. We wanted to capture a feeling of the conversations we've had with our friends in health, social care and on the autism spectrum whose thoughts and ideas have broadened our own views and understanding of the subject matter.

"The worst thing about death is the unexpected nature of it. If I was diagnosed with a life-limiting illness I would be able to plan what I wanted to achieve before I go."
(Person on the autism spectrum)

"I'm scared of using the word death. I feel I'd be putting a fear of loss in someone without being able to give them something concrete, something tangible to help them understand what I was telling them."
(Care staff)

"I think there is a lack of training for doctors in communicating with their patients. When you lack confidence in your ability to understand a patient with autism or a learning disability it's safer to retreat into your own area of expertise, back into your comfort zone of what you know."
(Doctor)

"It can be hard to take a step back and look after your own wellbeing sometimes, particularly at times where there are extra worries and pressures and you want to get things right for the person and their family. I would find the emotions of the families difficult, I'm not a trained counsellor."
(Care staff)

"It's easy for professionals to become precious about their own area of specialism and it's important to open ourselves up to the knowledge and insights of others."
(Community learning disability nurse)

"We've started to build some partnership working between us as a care provider and our local hospice and healthcare teams. It's been important to share training and knowledge, to start building relationships that will help us plan routes for joint working in the future."
(Social care manager)

"My worry is around how we get a diagnosis quickly enough for patients on the autism spectrum who struggle to communicate symptoms or are fearful of appointments and engaging with health staff. Those problems could have very serious consequences for someone's health and prognosis.

For people who are dependent on carers to advocate for them in healthcare consultations, they require support from someone who is strong and knowledgeable about that person to push for further investigations. I find it's worth going along to a consultation prepared with notes and observations."
(Care staff)

"I am a doctor working in hospice care that has never once worked with or known a person with autism. In mainstream services I feel we lack experience and knowledge of how to support people who have some very different needs to what we're used to."
(Doctor)

"I have a sister who has autism and severe communication difficulties and I'm scared that someone could take important decisions about her treatment who doesn't know or understand her. I worry about other people making presumptions about her quality of life."
(Family member)

"My hope is that integration of health and social care services should result in a more holistic approach to managing serious and life-limiting illness for those with autism and learning disabilities."
(Learning disability liaison worker)

"I think it's hard to give someone you support bad news, you worry about putting extra worry on them, particularly when you work with someone who experiences anxieties about so much in life. You know that stress has an effect on their general health already without adding to that. I think that's a big responsibility and I would like support if I had to do that from learning disability and speech and language teams to get my communication right."
(Care staff)

"It's about respecting each person's individuality, and within that their autism, recognising that is part of who they are and how they think and what is important within their life."
(Care staff)

"I was involved in supporting someone with autism at the end of their life. Sometimes the challenges of their autism affected my ability to accurately assess as I would normally do. I was unsure of what resources were available to support a patient with autism and the patient didn't have any other agency involved other than primary care."
(Palliative care clinical nurse specialist)

"It is interesting because even though it isn't clear from the research I've carried out whether care homes are solely catering to autistic people or whether a wide range of care homes have undergone specific training to understand the needs of autistic people at a time where they may be at their most vulnerable, the thought of tailored support is something that can surely only be a good thing for anybody who requires it."
(Person on the autism spectrum)

"The key to anyone's palliative care is to listen to those who know them best, often a closest relative. It is helpful to know that there is support available for professionals from other agencies and organisations."
(Palliative care community nurse specialist)

"I imagine having to work through a situation like Stephane's would change how I prioritised looking at the dreams and aspirations of the people I supported."
(Care staff)

"The team I manage had to cope with the death of someone we were supporting. It was difficult to describe how I felt at the time. I felt plastic, that was the only word I could use to describe it. Hollow and plastic. It was a horrible feeling but as the manager of a grieving team I felt that I had to be strong for us all.

We kept in contact with the family for a while but then after a year or so had passed they didn't get in touch anymore. That was sad too, but people get on with their lives."
(Social care manager)

"I remember having a conversation with a family about what they wanted to happen if something happened to them or their daughter. I was worried about whether or not it was the right thing to do. But I was glad we were brave enough to have that conversation because they were very sure about their wishes and had clearly thought about it before. I suppose lots of us think about these kinds of things but we don't want to share them or think about letting people know our wishes."
(Social worker)

"It's important to be clear about who takes responsibility for making important decisions, particularly where the patient may or may not be able to make decisions; to be clear about the role of the doctor, the family, the care staff and how we listen to the person themselves at such an important time."
(Care staff)

"It's a difficult job for a GP or clinician who is basing their course of action on what has been said in the consultation. That's why it's important to build good relationships with GPs and primary care staff. A lot of health professionals are working in highly specialised fields, but they're not specialising in autism. It's our job to bridge that gap."
(Social care manager)

"A lot of the fears for people with autism are the same as they are for you or me. Poor experiences of NHS care or treatment affect how we all feel about the future. These are common fears we can all relate to, particularly at the end of life."
(Community palliative care nurse)

Final thoughts

Stephane's story

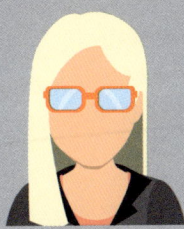

Valerie
Manager

"I felt like we were in a bubble for that period. I didn't realise until afterwards how focused we were on Stephane's care. So much so that when we did come out the other side it felt like we had emerged, emerged a much stronger and more knowledgeable team."

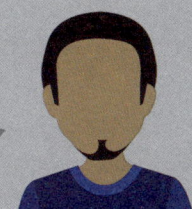

Justin
Support worker

"I just thought how would I like to be treated if I only had a limited amount of time to live. We just did the best we could and I hope we did well for Stephane. I think it's hard to realise what's happening till it's over sometimes, and you can go back and reflect on what we did well, what we could have done differently, what would we have wanted or needed to know. Hopefully by doing this now we can do a little to help other care teams who may find themselves supporting someone at the end of their life."

"Palliative care begins from the understanding that every patient has his or her own story, relationships and culture and is worthy of respect as a unique individual."

(Saunders, in Higginson et al 2004)

Whoever we are and regardless of our age, ability or cultural background the process of ageing and the inevitability of death is the common thread that runs through all our lives. The themes of physical, social, psychological and spiritual support inform our sense of self, of relatedness and of personal meaning in life. Identifying what is important to us comes never more to the fore than when faced with our own mortality.

For people on the autism spectrum – who can struggle to access equitable healthcare, whose social communication and understanding difficulties may affect how they form and sustain a network of social support, whose differing perspectives and thinking styles may affect the way they understand their illness and express how they feel and whose sense of spirituality may involve a deeply personal yet fragmented sense of selfhood and perceptual experience – there is a requirement for support and accommodations from diagnosis through to the end of life that are particularly person centred and inclusive of the diversity of needs in a broad and varied spectrum of individuals.

In light of the barriers to medical assessment and treatment highlighted for people with communication difficulties and learning disabilities in reports such as *Death by Indifference* (Mencap, 2007) and *The Confidential Inquiry into the Deaths of People with Learning Disabilities* (Heslop et al, 2013), it is all the more imperative we take a proactive and preventative approach to the management of healthcare needs for people on the autism spectrum throughout their life. This can help ensure that preventable and hidden illnesses are addressed where possible for those individuals who struggle to find a voice in consultations and articulate their symptoms.

The Disability Rights Commission (2006) highlighted that people with a learning disability, and therefore a significant percentage of people on the autism spectrum with learning and communication difficulties, are four times more likely to die of a treatable illness in large part due to delays in treatment and diagnosis.

In *Living and Dying With Dignity* (Morris and Read, 2008) the AWARE checklist reminds carers of their role in championing early intervention and better healthcare for the people they support:

- **A**lert people to the potential for ill health
- **W**atchful and vigilant for signs of ill health and change
- **A**ttend regular screening programmes
- **R**emember to encourage people to tell someone if they don't feel well or notice changes in their body
- **E**ncourage and enable people to attend appointments and understand the benefits of doing so

Conversations surrounding our death are about recognition of what is important in life and shouldn't wait for a diagnosis of a life-limiting illness or the planning of a funeral. The quest for wellbeing and fulfilment in life recognises the holistic interaction, throughout life and not just in the face of death, of our physical health, social relationships, psychological and spiritual needs. Having discussions with individuals and their families about future wishes prior to a traumatic event such as an unexpected death can enable all those involved to have a better understanding of everyone's wishes and expectations without having to explore them at a time of heightened emotion and distress.

It is understandable that amidst the pressures and considerations of day-to-day life we are not keen to stop and contemplate our death and the deaths of those we know and support. Future planning can be especially difficult for families and carers who are coping with some of the general pressures of supporting an individual with complex support needs (Towers, 2013).

Helping someone to set out their wishes for the future in conjunction with the people who are important to them, and supporting them to live a fulfilled and meaningful life in the time that they have, are the only ways we can minimise the distress of the death of a person on the autism spectrum we know or support. Person centred planning and engagement should be proactive and capture what is important in the person's life so that no one is left with feelings of regret or distress. People should be able to celebrate the happiness, fulfilment and achievements from the person's life.

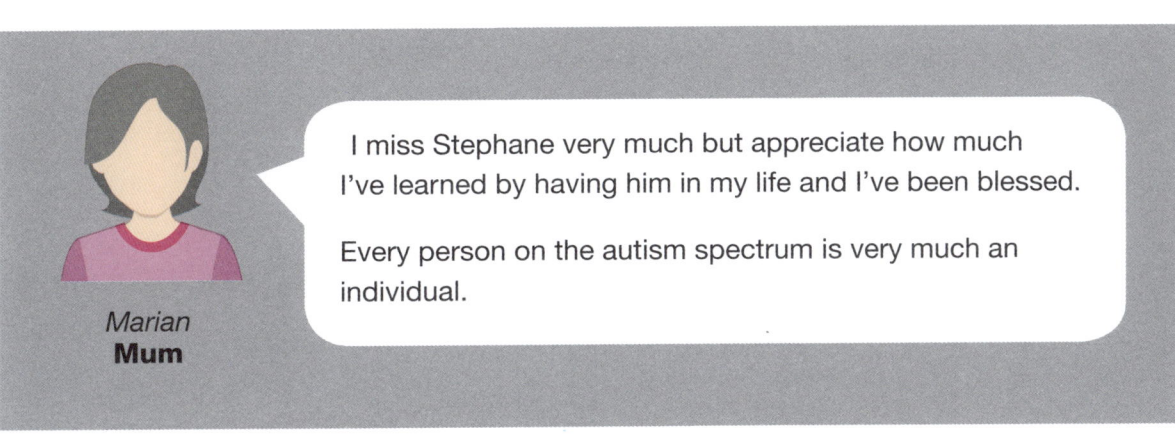

Marian **Mum**

I miss Stephane very much but appreciate how much I've learned by having him in my life and I've been blessed.

Every person on the autism spectrum is very much an individual.

Phil Evans is a freelance writer whom we met at a conference where we were sharing the video clips of the team discussing their experiences supporting Stephane. Phil is on the autism spectrum himself and was interested in talking to us about our experiences. He offered to contribute his own thoughts to this book:

> *"Autism isn't a physical difference. It's something that cannot be seen and as a result, it's something a lot of people can fail to pick up on or understand. As a person with autism myself, I've faced a lot of obstacles and have changed the way I've thought about or reacted in a situation to bring a positive result. I've been lucky in finding a way to adapt situations to my strengths. If I was facing the need for end of life care, however, I would need support from people I have a friendship and bond with to get through a difficult time. In a situation where incredibly raw feelings may need to be dealt with that may not present as neurotypical or 'normal', I'd want to put my trust in people who understand the nuances of autism and end of life care. Not somebody who knew one or the other."*

(Evans, 2015)

A need for stronger links between health and social care services for people on the autism spectrum is essential if we are to provide holistic end of life care that encompasses a developed understanding of the person's individual needs.

The National Council for Palliative Care's manifesto highlights three key principles in palliative and end of life care planning:

> *That everyone has a right to palliative care services as appropriate to their need*
>
> *That everyone should be able to exercise choice about their place of care at end of life*
>
> *That everyone is entitled to a good death*

(National Council for Palliative Care, 2005)

There is a gap which needs to be bridged between social care staff who have no experience of supporting someone's physical care needs and healthcare professionals with little knowledge of supporting people on the autism spectrum. A commitment to sharing knowledge and learning and working together to achieve 'a good death', will help to provide the best possible outcome for the person at the centre of that care and support.

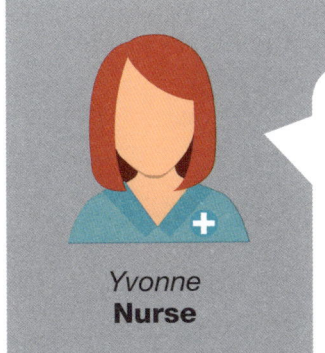

Yvonne
Nurse

The last thing we want for someone's final days is for them to be frightened, to be without comfort and peace. That's why it's so important we work together to get it right for individuals like Stephane.

I think it's because I have a son with autism that it makes me feel reassured that we can do this. Because you never know what the future will bring, and if that ever happened to my son I feel reassured that he'll be OK.

"

Pause for thought…

Our understanding of the autism spectrum is continually developing in the light of new knowledge and the shared experiences of those on the autism spectrum and the people who know and support them.

"Knowledge is not predefined or 'out there', but continually changing in the light of new experiences."

(Drumm, 2013)

D'Astous and colleagues recognise the interconnection of scientific development, social awareness and service provision in the historical narrative of support for people on the autism spectrum (D'Astous et al, 2014). As many of the children first diagnosed with autism now progress through to middle and older age and advances in autism awareness lead to an increased prevalence of diagnosis for older individuals on the autism spectrum, there will be an increasing emphasis on looking to the future. As we explore the individual narratives and life trajectories of the people we know and support, their experiences will influence and help shape the scientific, social and service contexts of current and future support.

This practitioner resource originated from a team of people willing to share a story so that we can develop our knowledge and understanding in a way that helps us prepare for the future. The important people in his life were devastated by Stephane's diagnosis and prognosis and had never before stopped to think about palliative and end of life care for a person on the autism spectrum they support. Even in the face of challenging and often upsetting experiences there is knowledge and insight to be gained and a realisation that *"dying is still a part of living"* (Wright, 2007).

There will be few occasions in life like the diagnosis of life-limiting illness that will throw life's priorities and meanings to the fore of

Final thoughts

discussions. Autism at its core is about human experience and exploration of themes of physical, psychological, social and spiritual support towards the end of life requires an insight into the breadth of human experience encapsulated by the rich spectrum of people with a diagnosis of autism.

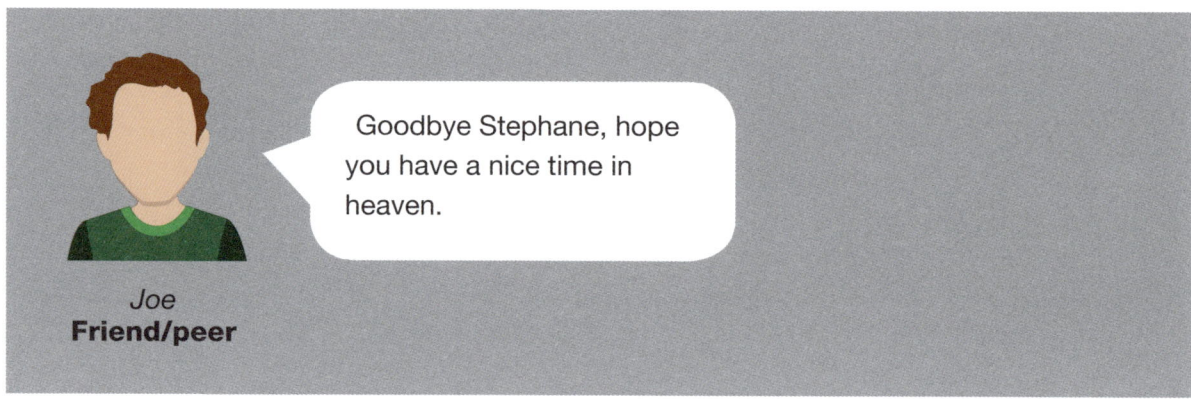

Joe
Friend/peer

"Goodbye Stephane, hope you have a nice time in heaven."

Information and support

British Institute of Learning Disabilities (BILD)

Advice and information for people with learning disabilities, professionals, families and carers.

www.bild.org.uk

www.bild.org.uk/information/ageingwell

Dying Matters

A coalition with the aim of encouraging open conversations about issues relating to death and dying.

www.dyingmatters.org

Foundation for People with Learning Disabilities

National charity working to improve the lives of people with a learning disability.

www.learningdisabilities.org.uk

Hospice UK

Hospice UK is the national charity for hospice care, supporting hospices to deliver the highest quality of palliative care to people with terminal or life-limiting illness.

www.hospiceuk.org

Macmillan

Macmillan Cancer Support offers information, support and advice for people with a cancer diagnosis and their carers.

www.macmillan.org.uk

Marie Curie

Marie Curie provide guidance and support for people diagnosed with a terminal illness.

www.mariecurie.org.uk

Mencap

Mencap are an organisation that work in partnership with and campaign for the rights of people with learning disabilities.

www.mencap.org.uk

The National Council for Palliative Care (NCPC)

The National Council for Palliative Care provides publications, downloadable resources and policy information regarding end of life for England, Wales and Northern Ireland.

www.ncpc.org.uk

PCPLD (Palliative Care for People with Learning Disabilities) Network

The PCPLD Network raise awareness of the palliative care needs of individuals with learning disabilities through the sharing of resources and best practice.

www.pcpld.org

Scottish Autism

Scottish Autism provides support dedicated to enriching the lives of people with autism through the whole life journey.

www.scottishautism.org

Scottish Partnership for Palliative Care

The Scottish Partnership for Palliative Care was set up to contribute to the development and strategic direction of end of life care in Scotland.

www.palliativecarescotland.org.uk

References

Abbey, J, De Bellis, A, Piller, N, Esterman, A, Giles, L, Parker, D and Lowcay, B (1998-2002) *Abbey Pain Scale*. Funded by the JH and JD Gunn Medical Research Foundation 1998-2002

Allison, H Green (2001) *Support for the Bereaved and Dying in Services for Adults with Autistic Spectrum Disorders*. London: National Autistic Society

American Psychiatric Association (2013) *Diagnostic and Statistical Manual of Mental Disorders: DSM 5 (5th edition)*. Arlington, VA: American Psychiatric Publishing

Baker, C and Wong, D (2009-2015) *Wong-Baker FACES*. Oklahoma City, OK: Wong-Baker Faces Foundation. Available to download at http://wongbakerfaces.org

Baranger, A and Sullings, N (2013) *Towards a Better Quality of Life: the rights of aging people with autism*. Brussels: Autism Europe

Baron, M G, Groden, J, Groden, G and Lipsitt, L P (eds) (2006) *Stress and Coping in Autism*. New York: Oxford University Press

Beresford, P, Adshead, L and Croft, S (2006) *Palliative Care, Social Work and Service Users: Making Life Possible*. London: Jessica Kingsley Publishers

Blackman, N (2003) *Loss and Learning Disability*. London: Worth Publishing

Blackman, N (2008) The development of an assessment tool for the bereavement needs of people with learning disabilities. *British Journal of Learning Disabilities,* 36 (3), 165–170

Blackman, N and Todd, S (2005) *Caring for Dying People with Learning Disabilities: A practical guide for carers*. London: Worth Publishing

Boerner, K, Burack, O, Jopp, D and Mock, S (2015) Grief after patient death: direct care staff in nursing homes and homecare. *Journal of Pain and Symptom Management,* 49(2), 214–222

Bogdashina, O (2011) *Autism and the Edges of the Known World: Sensitivities, language and constructed realities*. London: Jessica Kingsley Publishers

Bogdashina, O (2013) *Autism and Spirituality: Psyche, self and spirit in people on the autism spectrum*. London: Jessica Kingsley Publishers

Bolton, G (2008) *Dying, Bereavement and the Healing Arts*. London: Jessica Kingsley Publishers

Bond, C, Lavy, V and Wooldridge, R (2008) *Palliative Care Toolkit: Improving care from the roots up in resource-limited settings*. London: The Worldwide Palliative Care Alliance/ Help the Hospices

Booth, B, McDonald, F, Gower, D, Harrison, T and Kennedy, J (2010) *Palliative Care, End of Life Care and Bereavement*. CHANGE Cancer Series. Leeds: CHANGE

British Medical Association (2015) *Focus on Anticipatory Prescribing for End of Life Care*. London: British Medical Association. Available to download at http://bma.org.uk

Brown, L and Walter, T (2014) Towards a social model of end-of-life care. *British Journal of Social Work,* 44(8), 2375-2390

Buchsbaum, B C (1996) Remembering a parent who has died: a developmental perspective. In D Klass, P S Silverman, and S L Nickman (eds), *Continuing Bonds*. Philadelphia, PA: Taylor and Francis

Caldwell-Harris, C, Fox Murphy, C, Velazquez, T and McNamara, P (2011) *Religious Belief Systems of Persons with High Functioning Autism.* Boston, MA: Boston University

Charlton, R and Happe, F (2012) Aging in autism spectrum disorders: a mini review. *Gerontology,* 58(1), 70–78

Clements, J and Zarkowska, E (2000) *Behavioural Concerns and Autistic Spectrum Disorders: Explanations and strategies for change.* London: Jessica Kingsley Publishers

Community Learning Disability Team (2013) *What If: Celebrating my life. North East Lincolnshire NHS.* Available to download at http://www.pcpld.org

Corcoran, P, Nte, S, Read, S and Stephens, R (2011) *PicTTalk: A pictorial tool for talking.* Available to download at http://www.keele.ac.uk/nursingandmidwifery/research/picttalk

Cross, H, Cameron, M, Marsh, S and Tuffrey-Wijne, I (2012) Practical approaches toward improving end-of-life care for people with intellectual disabilities: effectiveness and sustainability. *Journal of Palliative Medicine,* 15(3), 322–326

D'Astous, V, Manthorpe, J, Lowton, K and Glaser, K (2014) Retracing the historical social care context of autism: a narrative overview. *British Journal of Social Work,* 2014, 1–19. doi:10.1093/bjsw/bcu131

Davies, E and Higginson, I J (2004) *Palliative Care: The solid facts.* Copenhagen: World Health Organisation

Department of Health (2006) *Introductory Guide to End of Life Care in Care Homes.* NHS End of Life Care Programme. Leicester: The Department of Health

Disability Rights Commission (2006) *Equal Treatment: Closing the gap.* Available to download at http://disability-studies.leeds.ac.uk

Drumm, M (2013) *IRISS Insights 23: The role of personal storytelling in practice.* Glasgow: Institute for Research and Innovation in Social Services

Dying Matters (2015) *Being with Someone When They Die.* Available to download at http://www.dyingmatters.org

Faherty, C (2008) *Understanding Death and Illness and What They Teach about Life: An interactive guide for individuals with autism or asperger's and their loved ones.* Arlington, TX: Future Horizons

Faull, C, de Caestecker, S, Nicholson, A and Black, F (2012) *Handbook of Palliative Care.* Hoboken, NJ: Wiley-Blackwell

Forrester-Jones, R and Broadhurst, S (2003) *Autism and Loss.* London: Jessica Kingsley Publishers

Foundation for People with Learning Disabilities (2015) *Learning Disabilities Statistics: Autism.* Available to download at http://www.learningdisabilities.org.uk

Garland, T (2014) *Self-Regulation Interventions and Strategies.* Eau Claire, WI: PESI Publishing and Media

Gawande, A (2014) *Being Mortal: Illness, medicine and what matters in the end.* London: Profile Books/Wellcome Collection

General Medical Council (2010) *Treatment and Care Towards the End of Life: Good practice in decision making.* Manchester: General Medical Council

Gerland, G (2013) *Secrets to Success for Professionals in the Autism Field: An insider's guide to understanding the autism spectrum, the environment and your role.* London: Jessica Kingsley Publishers

Hatton, C, Turner, S, Shah, R, Rahim, N and Stansfield, J (2004) *Religious Expression, A Fundamental Right: The report of an action research project on meeting the religious needs of people with learning disabilities.* London: Foundation for People with Learning Disabilities/ Mental Health Foundation

Henry, C and Ryder, S (2008) *Advance Care Planning: A guide for health and social care staff.* Leicester: Department of Health

Henry, C, Hayes, A, Holloway, M, Smith, T, Sherwin, E and Lindsey, K (2013) *Pathways Through Care at End of Life.* London: Jessica Kingsley Publishers

Heslop, P, Blair, P, Fleming, P, Hoghton, M, Marriott, A and Russ, L (2013) *The Confidential Inquiry into the Deaths of People with Learning Disabilities* (CIPOLD).Bristol: Norah Fry Research Centre

Hogg, M and Abrams, D (1988) *Social Identifications: A social psychology of intergroup relations and group processes.* London: Routledge

IRISS (2010) *IRISS Insights 02: Effectively engaging and involving seldom-heard groups.* Glasgow: Institute for Research and Innovation in Social Services

Isanon, A (2008) *Spirituality and the Autism Spectrum: Of falling sparrows.* London: Jessica Kingsley Publishers.

Jarrett, C (2014) Autism – myth and Reality. *Autism,* 27(10), 746–749

Jones, J (2002) *BILD Factsheet: Communication.* Birmingham: British Institute of Learning Disabilities

Jordan, R (2001) *Autism with Severe Learning Difficulties.* London: Souvenir Press

Kenny, L, Hattersley, C, Molins, B, Buckley, C, Povey, C and Pellicano, E (2015) Which terms should we use to describe autism? Perspectives from the UK autism community. *Autism,* 2015, 1–21. doi:10.1177/1362361315588200

Kim, C (2014) Acceptance as a wellbeing practice. In G Jones and E Hurley (eds), *Good Autism Practice: Autism, happiness and wellbeing.* Birmingham: BILD Publications

Kirkendall, A, Waldrop, D and Moone, R (2012) Caring for people with intellectual disabilities and life-limiting illness: merging person-centred planning and patient-centred, family-focused care. *Journal of Social Work in End-of-Life and Palliative Care,* 8(2), 135–150

Kubler-Ross, E (1973) *On Death and Dying.* London: Routledge

Lawson, W (2000) *Life Behind Glass: A Personal Account of Autism Spectrum Disorder.* London: Jessica Kingsley Publishers

Macmillan Cancer Support and Marie Curie Cancer Care (2013) *End of Life: A guide, a booklet for people in the final stages of life, and their carers.* London: Macmillan Cancer Support/ Marie Curie Cancer Care

Marie Curie Cancer Care (2015) *Changes in Breathing Towards End of Life.* Available to download at http://www.mariecurie.org.uk

McCreadie, M and McDermott, J (2014) 'Tuning in'… Client/ practitioner stress transactions in autism. In G Jones and E Hurley (eds), *Good Autism Practice: Autism, happiness and wellbeing.* Birmingham: BILD Publications

McKechnie, R C (2006) What does the literature tell us about death, dying and palliative care for people with intellectual disabilities? *Progress in Palliative Care,* 14(6), 255–259

Meikle, J (2012) Family of Down's patient sue hospital over DNR order. *The Guardian,* 13 September. Available to download at http://www.theguardian.com/society/2012/sep/13/downs-patient-hospital-dnr-order

Mencap (2007) *Death by Indifference.* London: Mencap

Mental Welfare Commission for Scotland (2011) *Right to Treat.* Available to download at http://mwcscot.org.uk

Milberg, A, Friedrichsen, M, Jakobsson, M, Nilsson, E, Niskala, B, Olsson, M (2014) Patients' sense of security during palliative care – what are the influencing factors? *Journal of Pain and Symptom Management,* 48(1), 45–55

Milton, D E M (2014) Fragments: Putting the self back in the picture. In G Jones and E Hurley (eds) *Good Autism Practice: Autism, happiness and wellbeing.* Birmingham: BILD Publications

Mitchell, A J (2012) *Emotion Thermometers Tool.* Available to download at http://emotionthermometers.com

Morgan, K (2006) Is autism a stress disorder? What studies of nonautistic populations can tell us. In M G Baron, J Groden, G Groden and Lipsitt, L P (eds), *Stress and Coping in Autism.* New York: Oxford University Press

Morris, H and Read, S (2008) *Living and Dying with Dignity: The best practice guide to end-of-life care for people with a learning disability.* London: Mencap. Available to download at http://www.mencap.org.uk/endoflifecare

Morton-Cooper, A (2004) *Health Care and the Autism Spectrum: A guide for health professionals, parents and carers.* London: Jessica Kingsley Publishers

Mowat, H and O'Neill, M (2013) *IRISS Insights 19: Spirituality and ageing: Implications for the care and support of older people.* Glasgow: Institute for Research and Innovation in Social Services

Munn, J C, Dobbs, D, Meier, A, Williams, C S, Biola, H and Zimmerman, S (2008) The end of life experience in long-term care: five themes identified by focus groups with residents, family members and staff. *Gerontologist,* 48(4): 485–494

Murray Parkes, C (1998) *Bereavement: Studies of Grief in Adult Life* (3rd edition). London: Penguin

National Council for Palliative Care (2005) *Palliative Care Manifesto.* London: National Council for Palliative Care

National Council for Palliative Care (2010) *Involving People with Personal Experience: Small is Beautiful.* London: The National Council for Palliative Care

NHS Scotland (2012) *A Guide to Good Practice in the Management of Controlled Drugs in Primary Care – Scotland.* Available to download at http://www.knowledge.scot.nhs.uk

Oswin, M (1991) *Am I Allowed to Cry? Study of Bereavement Amongst People who have Learning Difficulties.* London: Souvenir Press

Ramachandran, V S (2003) *The Emerging Mind: The BBC Reith Lectures 2003.* London: Profile Books

Read, S (2012) *When Someone You Know Has Died… People with learning disabilities supporting each other.* Keele: Keele University

Read, S (2006) *Palliative Care for People with Learning Disabilities.* London: MA Healthcare

Regnard, C, Gibson, L and Matthews, D (2006) *DisDAT Disability Distress Assessment Tool.* Newcastle Upon Tyne: Northumberland Tyne and Wear NHS Trust/St Oswald's Hospice

Regnard, C (2014) *Deciding Right: An integrated approach to making care decisions in advance with children, young people and adults.* Available to download at http://www.nescn.nhs.uk

Regulation and Quality Improvement Authority (2011) *The Disposal of Medicines in Nursing Homes: A guide to good practice.* Available to download at http://www.rqia.org.uk

Rehal, K (2013) End-of-life care. In National Autistic Society (ed.) *Ageing with Autism: A handbook for care and support professionals.* London: The National Autistic Society

Royal Pharmaceutical Society of Great Britain (2007) *The Handling of Medicines in Social Care.* Available to download at http://www.rpharms.com/social-care-settings-pdfs/the-handling-of-medicines-in-social-care.pdf

Ryan, K, McEvoy, J, Guerin, S and Dodd, P (2010) An exploration of the experience, confidence and attitudes of staff to the provision of palliative care to people with intellectual disabilities. *Palliative Medicine,* 24(6), 566–572

Ryan, K, Guerin, S, Dodd, P and McEvoy, J (2011) End-of-life care for people with intellectual disabilities: paid carer perspectives. *Journal of Applied Research in Intellectual Disabilities,* 24, 199–207

Scottish Government (2008) *Living and Dying Well: A national action plan for palliative and end of life care in Scotland.* Edinburgh: the Scottish Government

Scottish Government (2010) *Do Not Attempt Cardiopulmonary Resuscitation: Integrated adult policy.* Edinburgh: The Scottish Government

Scottish Government (2013) *The Keys to Life: Improving quality of life for people with learning disabilities.* Edinburgh: The Scottish Government

Steinberg, SM (2011) Cultural and religious aspects of palliative care. *International Journal of Critical Illness and Injury Science,* 1(2), 154–156

Supportive Care Register (2014) *Initial Pain Assessment SCR5, Gold Standards Framework.* Available to download at http://www.goldstandardsframework.org.uk

Swinton, J. (2001) Come all ye faithful. *Health Service Journal,* 20 December, 24–25

Swinton, J, (2006) Spirituality, suffering and palliative care. In S Read (ed), *Palliative Care for People with Learning Disabilities.* London: MA Healthcare

Tantum, D (2012) *Autism Spectrum Disorders Through the Life Span.* London: Jessica Kingsley Publishers

Thomas, K (2006) Community palliative care. In M Fallon and G Hanks (eds), *ABC of Palliative Care.* Oxford: Blackwell Publishing

Thomas, K (2011) *Time to face death head-on.* 20 May. Available to download at http://www.bbc.co.uk/news/mobile/health-13395211

Towers, C (2013) *Thinking Ahead: A planning guide for families.* London: Mental Health Foundation/Foundation for People with Learning Disabilities. Available to download at http://www.learningdisability.org.uk

Tuffrey-Wijne, I (2012) A new model for breaking bad news to people with intellectual disabilities. *Palliative Medicine,* 17, 55–62

Tuffrey-Wijne, I (2003) The palliative care needs of people with intellectual disabilities: A literature review. *Palliative Medicine,* 27(1), 5–12

Twachtman-Cullen, D (2006) Communication and stress in students with autism spectrum disorders. In M G Baron, J Groden, G Groden and L P Lipsitt (eds), *Stress and Coping in Autism.* New York: Oxford University Press

Twycross, R, Ross, J, Kotlinksa-Lemieszek, A, Charlesworth, S, Mihaylo, M and Wilcock, A (2015) Variability in response to drugs. *Journal of Pain and Symptom Management,* 49(2), 293–306

Vermeulen, P (2014) The practice of promoting happiness in autism. In G Jones and E Hurley (eds), *Good Autism Practice: Autism, happiness and wellbeing.* Birmingham: BILD Publications

Walter, T (1999) *On Bereavement: The culture of grief.* Buckingham: Open University Press

Watts, J (2009) *Death, Dying and Bereavement: Issues for policy and practice in health and social care.* Volume 11. Edinburgh: Dunedin Academic Press

Williams, D (2003) *Exposure Anxiety: The invisible cage.* London: Jessica Kingsley Publishers

Winkler, D, Farnworth, L, Sloan, S and Brown, T (2011) Moving from aged care facilities to community-based accommodation: outcomes and environmental factors. *Brain Injury,* 25(2), 153–168

World Health Organisation (2015) *The ICD-10 Classification of Mental and Behavioural Disorders: Clinical descriptions and diagnostic guidelines (Version 2015).* Geneva: WHO

World Health Organisation (2015) *WHO Definition of Palliative Care.* Available to download at http://www.who.int/cancer/palliative

Wright, B (2007) *Loss and Grief Workbook.* Keswick: M&K Update Ltd